T0296192

CAMBRIDGE PUBLIC HEALTH SERIES

UNDER THE EDITORSHIP OF

G. S. Graham-Smith, M.D. and J. E. Purvis, M.A.

University Lecturer in Hygiene and Secretary to the Sub-Syndicate for Tropical Medicine

University Lecturer in Chemistry and Physics in their application to Hygiene and Preventive Medicine, and Secretary to the State Medicine Syndicate

POST-MORTEM METHODS

POST-MORTEM METHODS

BY

J. MARTIN BEATTIE, M.A., M.D.

Professor of Bacteriology, University of Liverpool
Formerly Joseph Hunter Professor of Pathology, University of Sheffield

Cambridge :

at the University Press

1915

CAMBRIDGE
UNIVERSITY PRESS

University Printing House, Cambridge CB2 8BS, United Kingdom

Published in the United States of America by Cambridge University Press, New York

Cambridge University Press is part of the University of Cambridge.

It furthers the University's mission by disseminating knowledge in the pursuit of
education, learning and research at the highest international levels of excellence.

www.cambridge.org
Information on this title: www.cambridge.org/9781107418004

© Cambridge University Press 1915

First published 1915
First paperback edition 2014

A catalogue record for this publication is available from the British Library

ISBN 978-1-107-41800-4 Paperback

EDITORS' PREFACE

IN view of the increasing importance of the study of public
hygiene and the recognition by doctors, teachers, administrators and members of Public Health and Hygiene Committees
alike that the *salus populi* must rest, in part at least, upon a
scientific basis, the Syndics of the Cambridge University Press
have decided to publish a series of volumes dealing with the
various subjects connected with Public Health.

The books included in the Series present in a useful and
handy form the knowledge now available in many branches
of the subject. They are written by experts, and the authors
are occupied, or have been occupied, either in investigations
connected with the various themes or in their application and
administration. They include the latest scientific and practical
information offered in a manner which is not too technical.
The bibliographies contain references to the literature of each
subject which will ensure their utility to the specialist.

It has been the desire of the editors to arrange that the
books should appeal to various classes of readers : and it is
hoped that they will be useful to the medical profession at home
and abroad, to bacteriologists and laboratory students, to muni-
cipal engineers and architects, to medical officers of health and
sanitary inspectors and to teachers and administrators.

Many of the volumes will contain material which will be
suggestive and instructive to members of Public Health and
Hygiene Committees ; and it is intended that they shall seek
to influence the large body of educated and intelligent public
opinion interested in the problems of public health.

AUTHOR'S PREFACE

IT is now generally recognised that the diagnosis and scientific treatment of disease must be based on a sound knowledge of the pathological conditions present in the various organs and tissues, and that the skilled clinician should be able, at the bedside, to picture the exact state of the organs in the diseased conditions with which he has to deal. The science of bacteriology has made fresh demands on the clinician by establishing very definitely the causal agent of many of these pathological conditions, and making it important for him to be acquainted with these bacteria, their mode of action and their results.

Such knowledge can only be adequately obtained by careful work in the post-mortem room and, it is therefore important not only that examinations should be made in all possible cases but that systematic methods should be adopted in such examinations, whether made in the hospital post-mortem room by a trained pathologist or in a private house by a general practitioner. Every pathologist of experience knows how important facts, in any given case, have been overlooked either because of want of system or because they were not thought at the time to be important, and most of us have seen the statistician or the research worker in despair because of the inadequate and often useless records even of the trained pathologist.

The object of the writer has been to set before his readers a definite method of procedure, and such modifications of this procedure which may be demanded by special circumstances, and to emphasise the importance of attention to detail. The methods are based on his own experience as a hospital pathologist for nearly fifteen years.

LIST OF ILLUSTRATIONS

No attempt has been made to give details of morbid anatomy or morbid histology, but the more important lesions which are found in the organs are indicated, the methods for recognition and demonstration of these are given and the points which should receive special attention and special description are noted.

The book is essentially one of methods and it is intended that it should be used in conjunction with text-books dealing with pathology and bacteriology and not that it should replace any of these. Experience as a teacher and an examiner in Pathology has impressed upon me the necessity of a knowledge not merely of the methods for removal and examination of diseased organs but also, and even of greater importance, of the special pathological lesions which should be looked for in any given case. A thorough knowledge of both general and special pathology cannot be dispensed with if post-mortem examination is to have its full value, but the ordinary medical practitioner who is called upon to examine any given case will, I think, be helped considerably if he is made acquainted with the more important pathological conditions which he should be on the outlook for in any given case. In the later chapters an attempt has been made to meet this need: thus, if a practitioner is called upon to examine a case of suspected syphilis he will find the various important lesions in the different organs set out, and will be able, on the evidence of such lesions, to give a diagnosis; again, in a case of pneumonia, there will be no difficulty in diagnosis, but it may be important to find the causal agent and therefore the method of procedure is outlined as well as the secondary lesions which should be looked for.

Bacteriological methods have been dealt with briefly but, I think, in sufficient detail to be of value not only to the medical man who conducts the post-mortem examination but to the trained bacteriologist, in that he will get his material from suitable cases from the proper sites, and in a condition which will enable him to make complete and satisfactory examinations.

In an appendix I have given some of the more important methods for preservation of organs, and for their histological and bacteriological examination. These I hope will prove of value.

I have to express my indebtedness to Mr Robert Frost, of the Pathological Department of the University of Sheffield, for notes of some methods which he devised and for his assistance with the illustrations.

J. M. B.

March, 1915.

CONTENTS

CHAPTER I

GENERAL CONSIDERATIONS

The infrequent use of post-mortem examinations by the general practitioner, as an aid to the knowledge of disease, is due, in large measure, to the supposed difficulties and inconveniences of conducting the examination in a private house. These difficulties are, I believe, much exaggerated. Very few instruments are required and, with very simple precautions, hardly any trace of the operation may be left to alarm or to annoy the relatives and friends. In dealing, therefore, with these general considerations it will be convenient to discuss them under two aspects—firstly as they specially concern the *general practitioner* and, secondly, as they affect the *hospital pathologist*.

A. THE GENERAL PRACTITIONER.

(*a*)   The instruments required are as follows :

(1)   A *strong knife* with a blade about 2½ to 3 ins. in length, for opening the body, for cutting through the costal cartilages, for removing the organs and for cutting them up afterwards. For the latter purpose, a good table knife is very useful.

(2)   A *saw*—an ordinary joiner's or butcher's saw of small size is the most useful.

(3)   A *chisel* and a *hammer* of any type must be available, where the examination of the brain is required.

(4)   A pair of *blunt pointed scissors* to be used in the examination of the intestines.

(5)   A pair of *dissecting forceps* and a probe pointed bistoury are very useful but are not indispensable.

(6)   A *needle* and some strong *thread*—preferably not of a prominent colour—must always be available.

(b)   The other requirements are :

(1)   Two large basins with water for washing hands, instruments, etc.

(2)   A small bowl or a cup for scooping out any fluid which has collected, or which may collect, during the operation, in any of the cavities of the body.

(3)   A bucket or slop-pail for the reception of serous effusions, blood, or any waste material.

The operator should always see that he has an abundant supply of water in the room, some cotton wool or a sponge, and plenty of old cloths or paper.   If waterproof sheeting can be obtained, it should be utilised, especially in cases where the post-mortem examination is performed on the bed.   The body should, where possible, be removed from the coffin and placed either on the bed or on a table.   The bed and the floor must, as far as possible, be protected with old papers or the waterproof sheeting so that the bedding, the bed clothes, or the carpets shall not be stained with blood.   In cutting into the various organs, they should be held over the bucket, or over the opened body so that as little mess as possible is made.

When the examination of the organs is completed, all accumulations of fluid should be scooped or mopped out from the various cavities, the organs replaced, and the body sewn up with the greatest care : all traces of blood should be removed from it and the clothing carefully put on.   Before the doctor leaves, he or his assistant should see that all waste material (blood, etc.) is got rid of and that the instruments, vessels and table are thoroughly cleaned so that when the relatives enter the room they may see no traces of blood.   If these matters are carefully attended to the practitioner will soon find that his difficulties in getting permission to perform autopsies will be greatly lessened.

B. THE HOSPITAL PATHOLOGIST.

The post-mortem room :

The size of the room will depend largely on the size of the hospital to which it is attached, but it is desirable that, where possible, it should be roomy and particularly that it should be well lighted and well ventilated. Artificial light is always unsatisfactory, mainly because some of the less-evident pathological changes are rather obscured by it, and colour changes which are often of great importance are not distinctive enough. Therefore in choosing a site for a post-mortem room attention should be specially directed to the possibilities of obtaining plenty of light. A roof light is a great advantage, but where this cannot be got, large windows are essential. Unfortunately the glass has usually to be of a type which prevents anyone viewing the work from the outside, and this generally means a lessening of the light. It is of course necessary that artificial lighting should be used at certain times. The fittings should be so placed that a good light is available over the body, as well as over the table where the organs are examined. Equally important is the ventilation and, where the post-mortem room is not overlooked, windows which open widely are the most suitable means to employ. Very often however it is necessary to have both air inlets and outlets at various points. An extraction fan or some other form of air extraction apparatus should, where at all possible, be placed in the roof or in one of the walls.

The walls should be capable of being thoroughly washed and disinfected and a lining of white glazed tiles is therefore a distinct advantage—besides being an aid to the lighting of the room. The floor should be constructed of one of the various types of impermeable floor-material, and so laid that it can be thoroughly washed with a stream of water from a hose. The floor-material should be continued up on the walls for a distance of 4 or 6 inches and the angle between the two rounded off. This rounding off should also take place at the corners, so that there are no difficulties in the way of the easy cleaning of the room.

A plentiful supply of water is essential, and by means of a hose this should be available at any part of the room. In addition there should be a supply on or near each operating table, which should be at once available by the operator for washing the body, the various organs, the table itself, and particularly his hands.

Equipment of the Post-Mortem Room.

The post-mortem table should be about 7 ft. 6 ins. in length, about 24 to 30 inches in breadth, and the upper surface should be from 33 to 35 inches from the floor. It may be made of slate, of glazed fire clay or of marble, and the margins should always be raised above the general level of the table. The table should be so placed that there is a definite slope towards one end, and from that end the drainage should be arranged. The discharges may be run into a special cistern or cesspool where disinfection may be carried out before the contents are run into the ordinary drains. The table should be capable of rotation, especially in post-mortem rooms where teaching has to be done.

The sink should be shallow and should be at a convenient height for the worker. The water should be delivered to the sink both by a rose tap, 6 to 8 inches above the level of the sink and so arranged that the water can be brought to bear on every part of the surface, and also by a pointed nozzle which can be pushed into the intestines or other hollow viscus. This latter should be placed at the right-hand side of the sink not more than 1½ inches above its surface. Sloping upwards from the left-hand end of the sink—where the drains should pass off—there should be a table, either of waxed deal, of plate glass, or of porcelain, on which the organs can be cut. The drainage from this table should flow freely into the sink.

A bunsen-burner or a spirit lamp should be placed on or close to this table as well as near the operating table, so that in cases where bacteriological examination is needed, the sterilisation of needles or the searing of surfaces may be carried out without delay or without moving the organ to some other part of the room.

A few sterile tubes, sterile swabs, tubes of culture media, clean glass slides, a couple of platinum needles, a test-tube stand, a few sterilised pipettes with a narrow bore and an old knife, a spatula or a soldering iron for searing surfaces should always be available for every post-mortem examination. It is very desirable to have a laboratory in connection with the post-mortem room where all the usual apparatus (pathological and bacteriological) is available. A description of such a laboratory is beyond the scope of the present book. There should be in connection with every post-mortem room either a part specially set aside or a separate room in which there is a sink with hot and cold water and the ordinary appliances, where the operator can have his hands and arms, etc. thoroughly washed after doing an operation.

The Operator. The operator should wear an overall, preferably fastening at the back and having very short sleeves. Under this he should wear a waterproofed apron with a large bib. Many pathologists regularly wear gloves—either the thin ones worn by the surgeon or thicker ones with gauntlets. In my opinion the thicker ones not only interfere with the delicacy of touch so necessary to the pathologist, but they are also a hindrance to various manipulations. In the wearing of gloves, of whatever kind, there is a very obvious danger. A small puncture may not be detected, and through this the septic material gets to the hands, while the operator is quite unconscious of it, and thus for an hour or longer his hand is bathed in septic material and at the same time that hand is in a chamber where all the secretions are being retained, and in consequence the chance of infection becomes very greatly increased. Personally, I much prefer to do post-mortems without gloves, except extremely fœtid cases where the odour is retained for hours afterwards. No sane man will operate with unprotected hands if he has any open wounds, no matter how small, but if the hands are whole there is, I believe, little risk if they are kept thoroughly washed and no blood or secretion allowed to dry on them.

The doing of the examination near a stream of water I consider of the greatest importance, so that the hands can be kept almost continuously bathed. It is for this reason among others that I have urged the placing of water taps on or near the post-mortem tables and the rose taps 6 or 8 inches above the surface of the sink. It was the late Dr Alexander Bruce who first urged me to adopt this method and an experience of almost 15 years has proved its efficacy.

If the pathologist prefers to wear gloves in all cases or in any special case, the care of the gloves should be undertaken by himself and not left to a subordinate. The gloves should be thoroughly washed immediately after the operation and before they are taken off, and on removal should be placed for a few minutes in some antiseptic solution, thoroughly dried, powdered inside and outside with French chalk and put aside till again required. The use of gloves which are water-proofed on the outside only cannot be too strongly condemned. There may be a difference of opinion as to whether gloves should be worn or not, but there can be no question that there is a very grave danger in using gloves which cannot be thoroughly washed after use—or in using gloves which are not carefully attended to by the operator himself.

After the operation has been completed, the operator should wash his hands and arms carefully in warm water containing an antiseptic such as lysol, and afterwards in fresh warm water. It has been my practice to avoid the wearing of ordinary gloves immediately after a post-mortem examination, believing that the gloves produce an incubating chamber in which the bacteria are more likely to flourish than if they are fully exposed to the air. This custom may not have any scientific basis for its observance, for the short time in which a busy pathologist can keep his hands in gloves may not allow of much active proliferation of bacteria on his skin. At the same time, it may be of some value, and it is a duty of the pathologist to take every precaution consistent with the efficient performance of his work.

Shennan says, " The pathologist frequently notices that he is more liable to local infections after his return from a holiday, when he is presumably in the enjoyment of perfect health, and at such time he should be all the more careful to employ all means of preventing infection." With this I agree, but at the same time I would urge that full precautions should be taken at all times. The pathologist must take the risks of his occupation, but with want of care in any single case he may sacrifice his life, whereas, if he consistently carries out certain precautionary measures, he can greatly minimise the risk which is necessarily associated with his calling.

The Instruments required.

Cartilage knives. It is an advantage to have a few of these, and in selecting them I advise the choice of a rather wide blade. The blade should be strong and the handle made of wood, not of metal.

Scalpels. A few scalpels of various sizes are necessary.

Bistouries. At least two—a curved probe-pointed and a straight probe-pointed one should always be available. They are useful for many purposes but are specially valuable in opening the heart, in cutting the dura, and also in dividing the spinal cord during the removal of the brain.

A brain knife. The blade should be thin (not double-edged) about 2½ to 3 cm. in breadth and about 30 cm. in length. The handle should be of wood or, if of metal, it should be well grooved so that it may be held firm without any chance of slipping.

Forceps. At least two pairs of dissecting forceps are required. These should be strong with a fairly broad and grooved bite, and it is always an advantage to have one toothed pair.

Scissors. One pair of strong dissecting scissors with blunt points, and with a cutting blade of about 6 cm. in length ; a similar pair with sharp points ; a smaller pair with a cutting edge of about 4 cm. and having one blade probe pointed and a small pair with long (3 or 4 cm.), fine blades and with sharp points are desirable. These latter are extremely useful in opening up fine vessels, ducts, etc.

Bowel scissors. These should have one blade longer than the other—the longest being about 12 to 15 cm. The St Thomas's

Hospital pattern is very satisfactory, but in spite of some disadvantages I personally prefer the older form with the hooked end on the longer blade—the hook being at an acute angle to the blade and not too sharp (Fig. 1).

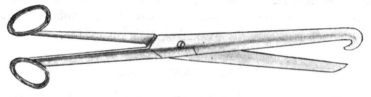

Fig. 1.

Chisel. The T-shaped chisel is the most valuable, though one of the ordinary chisels used by stone-workers is sometimes very useful.

Bone-forceps. These should be strong and it is generally an advantage to have the cutting parts and the handle set at an obtuse angle. The advantage of this form of forceps will be appreciated in the operation for the removal of the spinal cord. The two ends of the handles should be about 2 inches apart when the forceps are forcibly gripped in the hand. A second pair—the costotome—of the pattern shewn in Fig. 2 I prefer for rib cutting, etc. The lower blade is curved and blunt pointed. It can be passed under the ribs without the risk of any injury being done to the organ or tissues lying immediately behind the ribs.

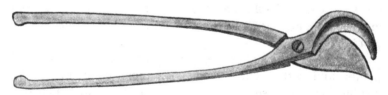

Fig. 2.

Saw. This should be strong and the distal end should be convex. A movable back, provided this fits tightly, is an advantage. In choosing take special care that the hole in the handle is not too small to admit the four fingers of the operator's hand. To be able to get a good grip of the saw is essential. For removal of the spinal cord I prefer a saw of heavy make such as that used by butchers.

Probes and catheters. Two or three probes of medium thickness should always be available, and in addition one or two metal or rubber catheters.

Mallet. This is always included in post-mortem sets, but it is really not essential. It should either be made of hard wood or of metal with a lead face.

Needles. These should be half curved and about 10 cm. in length.

Cord or twine. This should be strong and for preference of a light brown or greyish colour so that it will not shew prominently after the body is sewn up—which is always a consideration with the relatives.

Measures. A steel measure or measuring tape graduated both in inches and in centimetres, and a measuring glass in ounces and in cubic centimetres are necessary.

Balance and weights—ounces and grammes—should be provided. The hanging or spring balance is not so satisfactory as any of the ordinary forms of beam balance.

Several large wooden blocks—one grooved as a head rest—will be found useful for supporting various parts of the body during special operations.

In addition to the above, which should always be provided in a hospital post-mortem room, the following instruments are useful:

Lion forceps (for gripping the bones of the limbs or the vertebral column, etc. when removing these) ; *periosteum elevator* (particularly for stripping the periosteum from the base of skull) ; *grooved director* (for opening up ducts, etc.) ; *calipers* graduated in inches and in centimetres (Shennan's pattern I consider the most useful) ; a large *syringe* for removing fluid from the various cavities and a smaller one with nozzles of various size for injection of vessels.

Spine chisels, metal skull rests, coronets, double spinal saws, chain hooks, retractors and other instruments which have at various times been introduced are in my experience of very doubtful value, and certainly are not essential.

Cones for taking circumferential measurements, particularly of the valvular orifices, are still used by many pathologists and, if used with great care, they may give some information. By their use there is however the danger of destroying or rubbing off minute vegetations on the valves—vegetations which cannot properly be seen until the valve segments are fully exposed—and of the separation of recent adhesions. I have entirely abandoned the cones, partly on this ground and partly because I do not think the measurements of the orifices, obtained with them, of sufficient value to compensate even for the small amount of damage that they may cause.

It is important that all instruments should be kept thoroughly clean and in good order. Blunt knives and scissors are not only an annoyance to the operator, but they are also a source of danger. Greater pressure is required and if they slip the damage produced is often great. A very sharp knife is particularly important in the removal of the intestines.

Bacteriological Apparatus.

In case a bacteriological examination should be required the following apparatus should be at hand :

1. Half a dozen sterile cotton wool swabs, in sterile tubes.

2. A platinum needle.

3. A bunsen burner or a spirit lamp for sterilising the needles, etc.

4. A few sterile pipettes.

5. A searing iron. This may be a small-sized soldering iron or an iron spatula, or even an old knife.

6. A grease pencil for marking any tubes or slides.

7. An old scalpel, a pair of dissecting forceps, a pair of artery forceps and a pair of scissors, all of which can be sterilised in the naked flame, will be found useful in many cases.

8. A few tubes of sloped agar and also some bouillon.

9. Some clean microscopic slides.

10. A few sterile test tubes.

For special cases it may be necessary to have a supply of special media, *e.g.* blood agar, serum agar, bile-salt-lactose agar, etc., but where specialised examinations are required it is better to collect the material in sterile tubes and to make the more special cultivations in the laboratory.

Treatment of wounds. If the operator receives a wound, he should at once stop his work, and allow the cut to bleed freely under cold running water. The part should then be well sponged with some antiseptic solution and a carbolic compress put on. The practice of sealing up such wounds with collodion should be avoided. If it is necessary to continue the post-mortem the wound should be very thoroughly cleansed with an antiseptic, and a rubber glove which has been soaked in the antiseptic put on.

If at any time a small inflamed papule appears it is always advisable to treat it energetically and it has been my custom to cauterise it with a crystal of pure carbolic melted on the end of a straight platinum wire. With care the whole area can be destroyed and practically no damage done to the surrounding tissues.

Usually these simple precautions are successful in preventing the spread of the infective material and in averting danger ; but one cannot impress too strongly on the young pathologist that no matter how trivial the injury may seem he should treat it as if it were serious.

CHAPTER II

THE EXAMINATION

GENERAL FACTS.

Before the examination commences the pathologist must make certain that permission has been given for the operation by a legally responsible person. A pathologist may save himself a great deal of worry, and it may be the expense of a legal action, if he insists on having the written permission of some responsible person before he performs any autopsy. He should also have supplied to him the name and age of the subject, the day and hour of death, the more important facts in the clinical history and the clinical diagnosis. Too often these details are not supplied to the pathologist, and the value of the examination is thus greatly lessened. Such information is of value because it gives some indication to the pathologist as to the system he will adopt in conducting the examination, and calls his attention to those areas where special care is required. Owing to the necessary pressure of work it is often impossible to perform a thoroughly detailed examination in every case, and in many cases this is hardly necessary, but if the pathologist is not fully informed of the facts of the case important matters may be left uninvestigated. Most pathologists of experience will be able to recall cases where difficulties have arisen in the fuller investigation of the case because some organ or tissue had not been examined thoroughly. This difficulty would be minimised if proper records of all cases were supplied at the time of the examination. In a teaching hospital it is desirable that the physician or surgeon, under whose charge the case was, should be present during the operation, in order that the particulars of the clinical history may be given to the students, while the pathologist is doing the preliminary stages of the examination. No doubt the pathologist often discovers the errors of the clinician, but his object is and should always be to aid the clinician in finding out the true nature of the pathological changes which have been re-sponsible for the symptoms and physical signs observed during life. The true co-operation of clinician and pathologist must be mutually advantageous, and I cannot too strongly impress upon the young pathologist the advisability of encouraging this co-operation.

The post-mortem records. When possible the pathologist should have an assistant who takes manuscript notes of the case at his dictation. Sometimes however he has to trust his memory. In either case a record of the examination should be made as soon as possible after its completion, and at a later time this record should be added to as the result of more extended microscopical and bacteriological investigation. In many post-mortem rooms, printed record-forms are supplied to the pathologist. These have a certain value, in that the omission to note changes in any special organ is not so liable to occur as it is where no such form is used. This however is to my mind the only advantage among many disadvantages. With these set forms a certain space is necessarily allotted to a certain organ and, it may be, that in any particular case the main pathological changes are seen in that organ. The space is limited and the pathologist either has to contract his description, extend it into the space allotted to other organs, or disconnect it altogether.

The following is put forward as a suggestion.

Each record should be kept on a separate, numbered, double sheet of paper—about 12 in. × 8 in.—with a margin sufficient for binding, etc. At the top of the first page the following particulars should be printed:

POST-MORTEM RECORD. Number *x*.

Post-Mortem Diagnosis....................
Name.................... *Age*...... *Occupation*....................
Date and Hour of Death.......... *Date and Hour of Post-Mortem*..........
Physician or Surgeon...
Pathologist...

Note. Record the examination in the following order and if no pathological change is found in any particular organ or tissue, record this as " no obvious pathological change," or " not examined."

I. External Appearances : (a) Nutrition. (b) Colour. (c) Injuries or signs of disease, etc.

II. Internal Examination :

1. Thorax : (a) Pleuræ. (b) Pericardium. (c) Heart and vessels. (d) Mediastinal tissues.
2. Abdomen: (a) Peritoneum. (b) Appendix. (c) Spleen. (d) Kidneys and Adrenals. (e) Liver. (f) Stomach and duodenum. (g) Pancreas. (h) Intestines. (i) Œsophagus. (j) Mesenteric glands. (k) Bladder with ureters. (l) Internal and external genitalia. (m) Vena cava and aorta.
3. Mouth and Upper Respiratory Passages : (a) Tongue. (b) Teeth. (c) Pharynx with tonsils and adenoids. (d) Larynx, trachea and bronchi. (e) Thymus and thyroid. (f) Submaxillary, sublingual and other cervical glands.

4. *Head :* (a) *Scalp.* (b) *Skull.* (c) *Brain and membranes.* (d) *Spinal cord and membranes.* (e) *Pituitary body.*
5. (a) *Bones.* (b) *Bone marrow.* (c) *Muscles.* (d) *Nerves.* (e) *Nasal cavities.* (f) *External and middle ear.* (g) *Orbit and eyes in special cases only.*
Histological Examination.
Bacteriological Examination.

The External Examination of the Body.

The length of the body and its weight should be ascertained. It is convenient to have a scale marked on the post-mortem table in inches and in centimetres, and the weight may be ascertained by any convenient form of balance either arranged in connection with the operating table or in some separate part of the post-mortem room.

By a general survey of the body, as it lies on the post-mortem table, important information may be obtained as to certain pathological conditions—*e.g.* curvature of the spine, deformities of hands or feet, joint disease, wounds, bruises or other gross pathological changes.

I. *General State of Nutrition.*

Note should be made as to whether the body is well nourished and well developed, or whether there is emaciation or excessive adiposity.

1. *Emaciation*, in a child, suggests starvation either by want of food or by improper methods of feeding, congenital syphilis or tuberculosis ; in an adult, it points to chronic wasting diseases, *e.g.* tuberculosis, diabetes or perhaps more commonly to malignant disease especially affecting the œsophagus or stomach.

2. *Adiposity* often indicates prolonged alcoholic indulgence and frequently is associated with over feeding and absence of exercise. In women it is more common, and in some cases it is merely post-menopausal and not associated with alcoholism. The condition must be distinguished from swelling of the tissues due to œdema or to emphysema. Only a very superficial observer can however confuse the two conditions.

kl.

3. *General anasarca* (œdema). This swelling of the subcutaneous tissues due to accumulation of fluid in them, may be general, but it is more commonly localised and will be again referred to in dealing with the external examination of separate parts. It is commonly due to nephritis, cardiac disease, chlorosis or other forms of disease where there is excessive transudation of lymph, due either to alterations in the blood or to obstruction of the venous or lymph channels. It is not uncommon in cases of septic poisoning. The œdema is indicated by the swelling of the tissues—the pale, puffy character of the overlying skin and the pitting on pressure. In well marked cases of *myxœdema* anasarca may be simulated, but the pitting is absent or is very slightly marked and the skin is dry and often scaly. The hair is also scanty all over the body.

4. *Emphysema.* It is not common to get general emphysema, though the condition may sometimes extend very widely and is generally a result of fracture of the ribs with associated laceration of the lung, though it may also be present in the post-mortem changes associated with certain gas-producing bacteria, *e.g. B. aërogenes capsulatus*, and as a sequel of rupture of an emphysematous bulla, or of a phthisical cavity. The crackling on pressure easily distinguishes the condition from œdema.

II. *Changes in the Skin.*

Colour. The skin may be pale with very frequently a slight yellowish tint, or there may be very marked lividity. Between these two extremes all gradations are seen—the pallor being present in one area, the lividity in another.

a. Lividity and cyanosis. The lividity is often very marked about the head and neck, though perhaps it is more common in the dependent parts, patchy over the lateral aspects of the trunk and limbs and not uncommonly absent over the dorsal aspect of the trunk. The lividity in the head and neck is very commonly the result of conditions which lead to interference with the thoracic circulation or to asphyxia. It should be noted, however, that if the head has been dependent, and not properly supported after death, the lividity may simply be mechanical and the result of gravity. The livid discoloration (*cyanosis*) so commonly seen on the head and neck generally results from diseases of the heart and large vessels, the lungs and the mediastinal tissues ; such as congenital heart disease, inflammatory or degenerative changes in the myocardium, or in the coronary arteries, aneurisms or tumours in the mediastinum, causing pressure on the veins, pneumonia, pleurisy, etc.

The true post-mortem *lividity*, which is best seen in the dependent parts of the body, is absent from points on which special pressure is exercised, *e.g.* over bony prominences such as the iliac crests and sacrum. At first pressure with the finger renders a livid area pale, simply by emptying the blood vessels of the area, but later, when decomposition has commenced, there is a diffusion from the vessels of the hæmoglobin with distinct staining of the tissues—and this cannot be got rid of by mere pressure.

In deaths from severe toxic poisonings, or acute septicæmias, this diffusion out of the hæmoglobin is an early process, and the majority of the superficial veins become mapped out very distinctly and are usually of a somewhat pinkish colour. This pinkish network on a body recently dead should always be a warning to the pathologist that his examination is attended with considerable risk. In these cases, the hæmolysis of the blood which has taken place during life accounts in part for the rapid diffusion out of the hæmoglobin.

Post-mortem lividity is not usually confused with bruising, but, if in any case there is a doubt, an incision should be made into the discoloured area. In the bruise the blood is found not only in the vessels but throughout the tissues, which are often pulpy and shew distinct evidence of mechanical injury.

b. Pallor. This does not give much information but may be indicative of anæmia, and in pernicious anæmia it is commonly associated with a yellowish, or even a brownish yellow, tint.

c. Other discolourations. In Addison's disease the brownish black colour especially of exposed parts is well recognised, and

a general brownish discolouration of the skin is characteristic
of hæmochromatosis or " bronzed diabetes." In silver
poisoning—" argyria "—there is bluish-grey colouration of the
skin of the head and neck, the chest where it has been exposed,
and the hands, due to a deposit of metallic silver immediately
under the superficial epithelium. Sooty-black nodes may be
scattered over the body in cases of diffuse melanosis ; in pernicious anæmia and in other diseases where emaciation is a
marked feature, *e.g.* in carcinoma and tuberculosis, an increase
in the pigmentation of the skin is common—the colour
generally being brownish, resembling sun-burn. In septicæmia
a yellowish colour is common, but this is frequently due to slight
jaundice. The definite yellowish or greenish-yellow colour of
obstructive jaundice from malignant disease or gall stones need
only be mentioned.

Pale areas, due to absence of pigment, such as are seen in
so-called leucoderma and in anæsthetic leprosy, should be
looked for. Tattoo marks, pigmented areas, the result of
inflammatory or ulcerative changes, should be noted, as should
scars of recent burns, blisters and old scars of wounds, etc.
In medico-legal cases it is of special importance that these
marks, scars, etc. should be accurately described and measured.

The presence of any skin disease, with an accurate description of its character and distribution—the presence, situation
and extent of hæmorrhages, and the position and general
appearance of new growths, sinuses, ulcers, etc. should always
be included in any report.

III. *Decomposition Changes.*

The period at which these become evident varies not only
with the temperature of the atmosphere, but also with the
condition of the body. In summer the changes are seen at
a much earlier period than in winter, and in patients who are
much debilitated by long continued disease the changes often
become evident a short time after death. As a general
rule they are first indicated by bluish discolouration of the
abdomen—the discolouration being due to the action of

sulphuretted hydrogen and sulphide of ammonium on the iron-
containing pigments of the blood and of the tissues. At later
periods the discolouration becomes more widely spread.

In addition, at a later period, a development of gas takes
place, which may distend the various cavities and find its way
between the layers of muscle and into the subcutaneous tissues,
producing subcutaneous emphysema. Putrefactive and gas
producing bacteria are found in great abundance in such cases.

IV. *Post-Mortem Rigidity* (Rigor mortis).

Rigor mortis, in ordinary cases, supervenes in from three
to six hours after death. It first appears in the muscles of the
head and neck, then in those of the upper extremities and passes
gradually downwards by way of the muscles of the trunk to
those of the lower extremities. It passes off in the same order
and has usually disappeared in from twenty-four to forty-eight
hours. It appears early in patients whose muscles have been
rigidly contracted by convulsions before death, *e.g.* in cases of
strychnia poisoning and in cases of tetanus, and also where
patients have died of long continued wasting diseases such as
cancer, pulmonary tuberculosis and tabes mesenterica. In
these cases, the duration of the rigidity is short. In some cases
of marked emaciation it may be so slight and so evanescent
that the condition is not observed at all. It occurs late in
sunstroke. The condition, from the point of view of the pathologist, is not of great importance, but in medico-legal cases
it may give an indication as to the time of death. There are
however certain points, especially in its effect on the internal
organs, which, unless they are remembered, may lead the
pathologist into error. The muscles of the heart, and those of
the stomach and intestines, as well as the skeletal muscles,
shew the rigor. On the heart, the effect is to cause contraction
of the ventricle and to give the impression that the patient has
died during systole, or even that the ventricular wall has become
hypertrophied. In the stomach the condition of " hour glass "
contraction is often simulated, and in the intestine " agony "
intussusceptions are produced. The stomach, in these cases

can be easily and completely distended with water and there is no evidence of thickening of the wall at the area where the contraction was evident. The intussusceptions can be readily relieved and there is no evidence of any pathological condition in the coverings of the wall of the intestine at the sites at which they occurred.

EXTERNAL EXAMINATION OF SPECIAL AREAS.

The general external examination usually takes a very short time, and should always be followed by a more detailed examination of special parts. These may be taken in any order, but it is convenient to commence with the head and gradually pass downwards. In a description it is necessary to point out all the more important changes that should be looked for, but the actual examination, in the majority of cases, will occupy not more than a few minutes.

1. *Head and face.* The general conformation of the head should be noted and if there appears to be special increase or diminution in size from the normal, accurate measurements should be made, the condition of the fontanelles carefully examined and the consistence and thickness of the bone, as far as these can be judged by external examination, ascertained. Thus valuable information may be obtained in cases of hydrocephalus, acromegaly, osteitis deformans, and leontiasis ossea, in which conditions, enlargement and other changes are present, as well as in cases of microcephaly, etc. Any localised elevations or depressions should be noted, and careful examination made as to their position, their size, their consistence and their other general characters. Incisions should be made into these parts, where this is deemed necessary. In this way sebaceous and dermoid cysts may be detected, and much information may be gained in relation to simple and malignant tumours of the various types—primarily and secondarily on the scalp or on the bone. The naked eye appearances of these tumours may indicate to the experienced pathologist their probable nature, but in the majority of cases a microscopical examination should be a routine procedure. The more experienced the pathologist

the less likely is he to give any opinion without the aid of the microscope. Depressions are usually due to old fractures, to recent surgical interference or to actual disease and particularly to syphilis. If, in examination of these areas, it is found that the bone is eroded and actual perforation has taken place, the probabilities of the case being syphilitic are very great. Softened patches ("cranio-tabes"), sometimes attributed to rickets, are in the majority of cases syphilitic in origin.

Depression over the fontanelles is usual in infants and prominence in these areas indicates increased intra-cranial pressure, and is usually well seen in cases of meningitis, cerebral tumours and hydrocephalus. Irregular elevations ("bosses," "Parrot's nodes") are sometimes found at the margins of the anterior fontanelle and extending along the sagittal and interfrontal sutures in cases of congenital syphilis.

Wounds and bruises of the scalp should be carefully examined, their position, size and general characters being noted, and it is important to compare their position with the site of lacerations of, or hæmorrhages into, the brain substance which may be found at a subsequent stage of the examination.

Conditions of the hair and scalp, giving evidence of the presence of diseased conditions such as myxœdema, alopecia areata, ringworm, favus, eczema, œdema, hæmorrhage, etc. should be noted, and where possible local causes searched for.

The *face* should be examined in the same systematic manner and special note made of any abnormal condition in the eyes, including the orbit, the nose and the external nares, the mouth and the buccal cavity, and the external ear and auditory meatus. Such conditions as facial paralysis, and facial hemiatrophy, are usually very obvious as is also œdema especially of the lower eyelids, associated with renal or cardiac disease.

Tumours are not uncommon about the face and when present their character, their situation and size should be ascertained. Microscopical examination of such tumours is essential, and at this stage a portion of the tumour should be put in preserving fluid.

Rodent ulcers occur mainly about the forehead, the cheeks or the side of the nose; epitheliomas on the lips or cheeks; cystic tumours about the neck (branchial cysts) or in the mouth (ranula). Other tumours such as sarcoma, osteoma and lipoma may occur in this region. Enlargements due to glandular changes, e.g. in tuberculosis, and in mumps, should be distinguished from actual tumours. Lupus may cause considerable scarring of the face and tertiary syphilis may shew itself by gummata on any part of the face, producing deep ulcers as well as actual necrosis of bone—nasal septum, palate, frontal bones, etc.

Hæmorrhage from the nose suggests a careful examination of the nasal passages and the base of the skull, but not uncommonly it is due to blood being squeezed out of congested lungs, by pressure on the diaphragm, exerted by the gas-distended intestines. Hæmorrhage from the ear, and especially when associated with escape of cerebro-spinal fluid, indicates fracture of the petrous portion of the temporal bone. The detection of pus in, or escaping from, the ear, leads the pathologist to search for middle ear disease, destruction of the roof of the tympanic cavity, thrombosis of the lateral sinus and abscesses in the tempero-sphenoidal lobe or in the cerebellum. Extravasations of blood in the tissue of the external ear (hæmatoma auris), are sometimes seen in the insane, or may arise from direct injury.

The *eyelids* may show evidence of xanthema or xanthelasma in the form of yellowish flattened or nodular growths, of trachoma or of scarring resulting from former attacks, eczema or other forms of skin diseases or inflammatory changes. Protrusion of the eyeballs may indicate exophthalmic goitre or, if unilateral, a tumour in the orbit. The arcus senilis, the presence of cataract, the condition of the pupils etc. should be noted.

It is specially important when examining the *mouth* to observe any scarring or staining which may suggest poisoning by corrosives of any kind. Injuries and abnormalities of the lips, the teeth, the tongue, the gums and the palate should be looked for. Herpetic eruptions, especially on the upper lip are frequent in cases of pneumonia.

2. *Neck.* Scars of operative procedure or of healed ulcers should be noted. In the middle line the main pathological

change is enlargement of the thyroid in goitre and its atrophy in cretinism and in myxœdema. Enlarged glands should be examined especially in relation to tuberculosis, lymphadenoma, leucocythæmia or secondary malignant disease. Congenital cysts, or fistulæ may be found, on account of abnormalities in the thyro-glossal duct, or in the closure of the branchial clefts. Perforation of the larynx is rarely seen and, when present, other signs of syphilis should be carefully looked for.

3. *The thorax.* The general shape of the thorax should be noted—the "barrel-shaped chest" of emphysema and of chronic bronchitis ; the narrow, flattened chest of chronic tuberculosis ; and the "pigeon breast" of rickets. Local bulging, resulting from enlargement of the heart during early childhood, is sometimes seen over the cardiac region, and is specially characteristic of some forms of congenital heart disease. This bulging should always lead the pathologist to examine the heart with the particular object of detecting evidence of congenital abnormalities. The "beading" of the ribs in rickets and the local prominence sometimes seen in cases of aneurism of the arch of the aorta are generally very obvious. Deformities of the lower part of the sternum—prominences or concavities—may result from the occupation of the individual.

In females, tumours of the breast, and involvement of the axillary glands, may be looked for. Note should also be made of scars on the thorax and particularly any evidence in these scars of recurrent malignant disease.

4. *The abdomen.* The presence of striae gravidarum, and the general tone of the muscles of the abdomen should be noted.

Uniform swelling suggests either a deposit of fat in the walls or an accumulation of fluid in the cavity. In the former, the walls feel much thickened, the prominence is generally most marked about the middle line, and the umbilicus is situated in a depression ; whilst in the latter, the walls feel very tense, the bulging is specially seen laterally, the umbilicus is flattened or even projecting and the skin is often smooth and glossy. When the accumulation of fluid is due to obstruction in the portal circulation, the veins on the surface of the abdomen are prominent and dilated.

The same stretched, glossy appearance with great swelling is seen in the abdomen of children dying of tabes mesenterica. Palpation however always reveals irregular areas of resistance, and in these cases the greenish colour of decomposition appears very early. The abdomen in such cases appears to be extremely prominent, because of the marked emaciation of the rest of the body.

Localised and irregular enlargement of the abdomen may be due to tumour formation in the underlying viscera ; distension of special areas of the intestine, e.g. the colon in Hirschsprung's disease ; enlargement of the liver or of the spleen ; more rarely, enlargement of the kidney, and enlargement of the uterus in pregnancy. Localised swellings may also be observed at certain orifices or potential orifices, e.g. the sites at which herniæ occur. Unilateral œdema of the lower part of the abdomen and groin may be associated with mediastinal tumours pressing on the azygos vein. The side on which the œdema appears may aid in the determination of the site of pressure. The presence of any fistulous openings, the situation, size and general characters of wounds or bruises should be carefully noted. Their age should if possible be determined, and, if inflammatory action or actual suppuration has occurred, bacteriological examination should be made of the fluid. Careful examination should be conducted to elicit if there is any connection between the wounds and the peritoneal cavity and, if peritonitis is present, an attempt should be made to find whether the suppuration in the wound was a primary condition or secondary to the peritonitis.

At this stage, it is advisable to examine in the male the penis and scrotum for any sign of injury, abnormality or disease. Tumours, chancres, discharge from the urethra, scars of old ulcers or results of operation wounds should all be noted and where necessary microscopical examination of discharges should be made. In the female, examination should be made of the vagina and urethra for inflammation, especially as to the presence of purulent discharge ; for any evidence of venereal warts or condylomata ; for ulceration ; for tumours or any other abnormality.

The posterior surface of the thorax and abdomen should now be examined with special attention to deformities of the spine, and the presence of bed sores, tumours, etc. should at the same time be noted.

5. *The extremities.* The more important changes to be noted in the limbs are rigor mortis, especially in the lower limbs, varicose veins, œdema, ulceration, pigmentation, deformities, disease in joints or in bone, such as tuberculosis, syphilis, tumour formation, etc., signs of old or recent injury and degenerative conditions such as necrosis and gangrene.

The œdema may be confined to the legs and feet or may involve the whole of the lower as well as the upper limbs. It may be unilateral. Where it is bilateral it is usually due to cardiac or renal disease, but may also be brought about by pressure on some of the large veins. Where unilateral, it may be the result of pressure on some of the veins ; or it may be due to interference with lymphatic return as is seen in the arm after some cases of cancer of the breast, especially where the cancer has widely infiltrated the tissues over the chest (cancer en-cuirasse). Brownish pigmentation is common around the scars of old ulcers, but it is also marked in the front of the tibia in men who have to work constantly in front of large fires. Diseases of the joints are observed merely by the enlargement or by deformities. Syphilis may show itself by ulcers, pigmented scars of old ulcers, and nodes on the tibia.

In cases of gangrene the obstructed or degenerated vessel should be sought, though in some cases, *e.g.* Raynaud's disease, no obvious obstruction or degeneration is found. In the gangrene of Raynaud's disease there may be little or no discolouration of the skin, which is however glossy.

Note should also be made of any local atrophy of the limbs, such as results from diseased joints or from hemiplegia, or any enlargement, such as occurs in acromegaly or elephantiasis.

CHAPTER III

THE OPENING OF THE BODY AND THE REMOVAL OF THE VISCERA

The body is placed on the table in such a way that the head hangs over the end and the skin of the neck thus becomes well stretched. The operator stands at the right-hand side (if he is right-handed) and, holding the cartilage knife firmly between the thumb and middle finger and with the index finger on the back of the blade, he makes an incision through the skin and the subcutaneous tissue. If the post-mortem examination is an unrestricted one, the incision should commence at the angle of the jaw and pass directly downwards as far as the symphysis pubis, curving round the *left* side of the umbilicus, but never cutting through it (Pl. I fig. 1). It will be found advantageous, at the commencement of the incision, to put the skin of the neck or the upper part of the chest on the stretch between the thumb and forefinger of the left hand (Pl. II fig. 3).

Over the front of the thorax the incision passes as deeply as the surface of the sternum, but over the abdomen it should not pass deep enough to injure the peritoneum. At the lower end of the xiphisternum, the knife should now be carried carefully through the peritoneum over an area sufficient to admit a couple of fingers. The index and middle fingers of the left hand are introduced into the opening, with the extensor aspects in contact with the viscera and the points towards the pubis, the abdominal wall raised from the underlying intestine and the knife introduced with its back to the internal organs. The opening of the abdomen is completed by cutting from within outwards. The recti are next divided laterally from their internal aspect close to their attachment to the pubic bones.

The sternal ends of the abdominal muscles on the right side are pulled upwards and outwards, and the attachment to the costal margin cut through with a sharp knife. By pulling further on these muscles and cutting with a long sweeping motion towards the ribs with the knife almost parallel with them, it is easy to separate the muscles from the thoracic bony case and, by continuing these incisions upwards the skin and subcutaneous tissues are reflected from the neck. When these incisions have been completed, the thoracic wall as far as the anterior limit of the axilla and the great vessels in the neck should be exposed. In the same order and to the same degree, the left side of the thorax and neck should be exposed. In emaciated subjects this reflection of the skin and subcutaneous tissue should be done with great care, to avoid buttonholing the skin.

During the progress of this work the degree of adiposity and any special characteristics of the fat as well as any degenerative or other changes in the muscles should be noted. Normally muscle is of a purplish-brown colour, and the most important degenerative changes tend to render it paler. Thus, in acute septicæmic conditions, there is a distinct pallor of the muscle and not uncommonly a softening of its fibres. In typhoid fever and in some other toxæmias the pallor is patchy in character and, on careful examination, it is found that the muscle in these areas has lost its striation and has become homogenous, and that in addition there is fragmentation of the fibres. This degeneration of Zenker is found particularly in the upper parts of the recti abdominalis.

There is pallor of the muscles in various forms of anæmia, and a yellowish tint may even be detected where fatty degeneration has become pronounced. A darkening of the colour is not of great significance but is often seen in old people dying of chronic wasting disease.

In the only case which I have seen of carbon monoxide poisoning, the muscles were almost pink in colour.

Other abnormalities in the muscular wall, such as bruises, wounds, suppurative foci, etc. should be examined and notes made as to their size and character.

In females, the breasts should be examined and cut into from the under surface. The main pathological conditions which should be looked for are:

(1) *Mammitis.* If this condition is present its nature and

Plate I

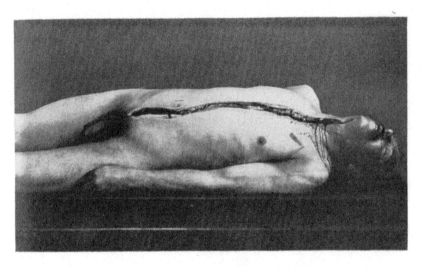

Fig. 1. Shewing the complete preliminary incision through the skin and subcutaneous tissues.

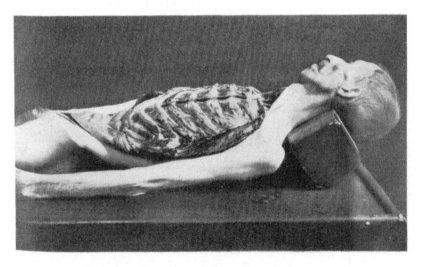

Fig. 2. Shewing the line of incision on the left side for the removal of the anterior wall of the chest.

extent should be examined. It will usually be chronic and shew itself by the presence of white fibrous tissue.

(2) *Tumours or cysts.* If these are present the naked eye appearances should be carefully noted and portions put aside for microscopical examination.

(3) *Purulent infiltrations* will always involve a microscopical and bacteriological examination for the causal organisms.

Thoracic walls. These should next be examined, noting particularly general alterations in shape, and local bulgings and local depressions. These latter can now be more accurately mapped out and their position more clearly defined than was possible from a mere external examination before the skin was reflected.

By this examination, evidence of rickets, fractures, infiltration and destruction of bones by tumour growth, deformity and erosion of bones by aneurisms is obtained. In addition the " beading " of the ribs due to the enlargement of the costo-chondral articulations is made more evident. The contents of the axilla should be examined at this stage.

Before opening the thorax the position of the liver and spleen should be noted and a general superficial examination made of the abdominal cavity for serous fluid or blood as well as for peritonitis, evidence of adhesions, intussusception, appendicitis or ulceration

Opening the thorax. Careless opening of the thorax may render uncertain the presence of pneumothorax. If such a condition is suspected, Shennan adopts the following plan : " A square is dissected out from the soft parts between the cartilages close to the sternum, so that the parietal pleura is exposed, and the hollow filled with water ; the pleura is then punctured. Air, if present, reveals itself by the escape of bubbles through the water." Usually when cutting through the costal cartilages the sound of escaping air gives sufficient indication of the presence of pneumothorax.

In opening the thorax, if the rib cartilages are not calcified, an incision is made on the right side, with the cartilage knife, in an oblique line passing downwards and outwards, just to the inner side of the costo-chondral articulations (Pl. I fig. 2). The knife is firmly held at an angle of somewhat less than 45° with the chest wall, so that when the distal part of the blade passes through the costal cartilages of the second rib the proximal part of the blade rests on the third cartilage. In this position the knife can be drawn quickly downwards and at the same time never penetrating deep enough to injure the subjacent lungs, even if these are adherent to the anterior chest wall.

In cutting it is generally advised that the edge of the knife should be directed outwards so that the ribs be cut through obliquely. Personally I prefer that the edge of the knife should be directed inwards, provided that the angle between the surface of the knife and the ribs is not less than 45°. My reason for adopting this method is that in fixing up the body at the conclusion of the examination the sternum fits into a depression which is narrower at the bottom than at the top, and the falling in of the front of the thorax is avoided.

The incision through the costal cartilage is made in the same manner on the left side.

The sterno-clavicular joints are opened from the front, care being taken not to pass too deeply, so that injury to the underlying vessels may be avoided.

The pathologist now pulls up the lower left cartilages, with his left hand (Pl. II fig. 4) and cuts through the anterior attachment of the diaphragm. The cartilages and the sternum are now pulled further upwards and with the knife held close to the under surface of the sternum and parallel with it, the remaining part of the anterior attachment of the diaphragm and the loose tissues connecting the sternum to the subjacent structures are separated (Pl. III fig. 5). This separation is very easily effected unless pathological conditions which have formed definite fibrous adhesions in this region are present. The concave blade of the costotome is next passed under the first rib: and the under surface of the sterno-clavicular joint on either side—the cutting blade extending through the opened sterno-clavicular joint above the clavicle (Pl. III fig. 6). By very slight pressure the tissues between the two blades are cut through and the sternum with its attached costal cartilages can be either turned to one side or cut away completely.

Plate II

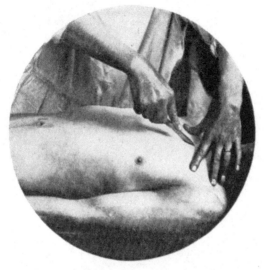

Fig. 3. Shewing the stretching of the skin, and the method of holding
the knife in the preliminary incision.

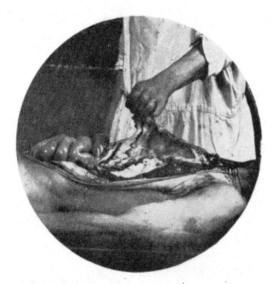

Fig. 4. Shewing the raising up of the lower part of the sternum and
costal cartilages previous to the division of the diaphragm.

If the rib cartilages are calcified, the safest method of procedure is to saw through the ribs in a line parallel with, and slightly anterior to, the anterior axillary line—the saw cut being extended through the clavicle. The sternum and its attached ribs are removed by the method already described. Bone forceps should not be used in this operation, as the ragged edges which they produce are a source of great danger to the operator.

Shennan recommends the following method in the case of young children, and I have found it of value :

" The customary median skin incision may be employed, or an incision corresponding to the line along which the cartilages on the right side of the body are divided. If the former be used then the soft parts have to be cleared off from the cartilages on the right side only. These are divided in the ordinary manner and the subjacent mediastinal soft parts separated from the sternum from below upwards and towards the left side. The right sterno-clavicular joint is next separated and the manubrium completely freed from the mediastinal structures. Still raising this "lid" as it were, one makes a hinge for it by cutting obliquely through the left rib cartilages and the left sterno-clavicular joint in the usual line, but from the under surface, the skin and soft parts over the cartilages being left uninjured. Quite as free access to the thorax is obtained by this method as by the one ordinarily employed, with the great advantage that the opening is easily and securely closed when the *sectio* is completed. It is difficult, otherwise, to prevent falling in of the sternum in young children."

Having exposed by any of these methods the thoracic and abdominal organs, careful note is made of any abnormalities or pathological conditions which are now observed in the costal cartilages, in the pleural and abdominal cavities, or in the thoracic or abdominal organs. In the costal cartilages the main point to be noted is the presence or absence of calcareous deposit. True ossification is a rare change. The pleural cavities and the peritoneal sac should be examined for fluid, but further details will be given on this point in the description of the examination of the thoracic and abdominal contents.

The Thoracic Contents.

A preliminary examination is made of the mediastinal tissues of the lungs and pleural cavities, and of the pericardium. *Mediastinal tissues.* These may be much thickened by œdema or by hæmorrhage, or there may be evidence of infiltration by new growths, especially by a primary lymphosarcoma. The thymus may be present and even enlarged. This gland which is a prominent structure in young children begins to atrophy about puberty, and from the ages of 21 to 25 it has almost completely disappeared. Much importance has been laid upon its enlargement as an actual cause of sudden death, or as a part of the general condition of " status lymphaticus " in which sudden death is said to occur. A discussion as to the merits of this question is beyond the scope of the present book, but one would strongly urge the young pathologist not to be satisfied with the diagnosis " enlarged thymus " or " status lymphaticus " as the cause of death. He may not have sufficient cause either in the clinical history of the case or in the post-mortem findings, but one feels strongly that " status lymphaticus " is very often a haven of refuge for the man who has not done an exhaustive examination, or who is not competent to judge of the effect of the findings which the clinical history and post-mortem examination have revealed.

Nevertheless, a knowledge of the general appearance, the size and the weight of the thymus is important to the pathologist. Normally its thickness is about 7 to 8 mm., and its breadth about 3 cm. In length it varies greatly in different individuals, and in weight it averages from 15 to 25 grammes. Narrow at the upper end it broadens out at its free extremity and the lobes, which are of a pinkish colour, almost meet in the mid line about half-way from the upper end of the organ.

The enlargement is generally shewn by an increase in thickness, breadth and bulk, and, as a general rule, if the organ exceeds the measurements given—which are probably slightly in excess of the average, it may be considered abnormal.

Plate III

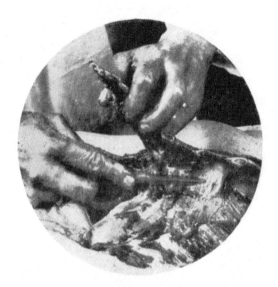

Fig. 5. Shewing the plane of the incision and the method of holding the knife in separating the sternum and costal cartilages from the diaphragm and the other underlying structures.

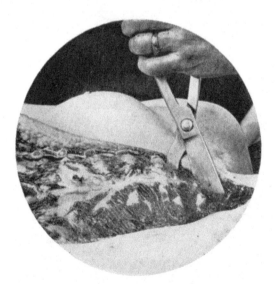

Fig. 6. Shewing the costotome in position in the division of the first rib on the right side.

Apart from the so-called " status lymphaticus," enlargement is sometimes seen in cases of leucocythæmia and not uncommonly in exophthalmic goitre.

Sarcomata may occur in the gland and, in cases of tuberculosis, caseous nodules have been found.

Any distension of the large venous trunks in the upper mediastinum should be noted and the cause looked for ; special attention being directed to such pathological conditions as tumours, enlarged glands, or aneurisms pressing on the superior vena cava or the innominate vein. In default of these conditions the explanation is usually to be found in the heart, where there is either valvular disease or degenerative conditions of the muscle.

The lungs and pleural cavities. The extent to which the anterior margins of the lungs overlap the heart should be noted, and any other points such as adhesions, the presence of inflammatory exudate, the presence of fluid in the pleural cavities. If there is fluid in the pleural cavities a small quantity should be withdrawn into a sterile tube before any handling of the organs and tissues takes place ; and any other condition suggesting the advisability of bacteriological examination should be dealt with at this stage. The details of the methods to be employed in bacteriological examinations are given later.

After this preliminary examination is completed, the hand should be passed carefully into each pleural cavity in turn, so that adhesions may be detected, their character and situation observed and then the adhesions should be broken across so that the lung on each side may be completely separated from the chest wall and from the diaphragm. Fluid accumulations should then be withdrawn, the amount of fluid measured and its characters observed—particular attention being directed to the presence of blood, of pus, or of flakes of lymph. Histological and bacteriological examination should be made of the fluid which has been previously withdrawn to determine the presence of red blood corpuscles, pus or other inflammatory cells, cells of malignant growths, fibrin, bacteria, etc. Blood-stained exudate indicates a very acute pleurisy or malignant infiltration of the pleura. It is however also found in some cases of tuberculosis, in infarction of the lung, in deaths from asphyxia, in severe septicæmias where there are numerous hæmorrhages in the pleura ; and in cases where there has been mechanical injury to the chest wall or to the lung. In the latter cases the blood may be in considerable quantity and may have formed soft easily broken down clots, a similar condition may result from the rupture of an aneurism into the pleural cavity.

The presence of polymorphonuclear leucocytes and fibrin in the exudate indicates that the infection has been recent. It must always be remembered that even large quantities of a serous fluid may collect in the pleural cavity during the few hours which immediately precede death, and that the presence of this fluid is not of special significance. In cases where the adhesions are very extensive and completely, or almost completely, obliterate the pleural cavity, it is generally more convenient to strip the costal pleura from the chest wall than to break down the adhesions—and in addition less damage is likely to be done to the lungs. In cases in which the pleural adhesions are marked only on the diaphragmatic surface careful search should be made for any pathological changes immediately below the diaphragm before the various organs are removed. In such changes as gastric ulcer, perihepatitis, abscess behind the liver, carcinoma of the stomach and old septic infarction or other disease of the spleen, the pathologist may find the origin of the adhesions.

Before the removal of the lungs the pericardium and the heart should be examined and removed.

THE PERICARDIUM AND HEART.

To open the pericardium. With a pair of dissecting forceps pinch up the most prominent part of the pericardial sac and make a small opening into it, and then with the curved probe-pointed bistoury continue the incision upwards to the base of the heart. If at this stage any evidence is seen of inflammatory or suppurative changes, cultures should be made from the exudate or fluid, selecting, of course, an area which had not become contaminated during the operation of opening the sac. If no special pathological changes are seen, or after the cultures have been made, an incision should be made from the middle of the previous incision and passing downwards towards the apex of the heart so as to open up as completely as possible the pericardial sac.

The presence of inflammatory exudate, of adhesions between the sac and the heart itself, of "milk" spots or of other pathological changes can be seen at this stage, and, in this examination, the dorsal as well as the ventral aspect of the heart should be carefully looked at and particular attention paid to the region of the great vessels, for it is very common to find inflammatory changes shewing themselves in this area alone. Petechial hæmorrhages, too, are frequently most marked in this region in cases of septicæmia.

If the exudate is hæmorrhagic, before the heart is removed careful search should be made for the presence of a ruptured aneurism in the region of the great vessels. Injuries to the heart itself, malignant disease, acute pericarditis, and rupture of the coronary vessels or of aneurisms on them, which may be responsible for the hæmopericardium, are best sought after the heart is removed from the body. Some of the blood or other fluid which may be found in the pericardium is taken in a sterile test tube, in case it should be afterwards required for histological or bacteriological examination, and thereafter the fluid removed and its quantity measured. The general shape of the heart, the condition of distension of the coronary sinuses and the amount of dilatation of the auricles, including the auricular appendices, should now be noted, for after removal of the heart the coronary sinuses become emptied, and the degree of auricular and ventricular enlargement is not so accurately judged. Examination of the aorta should be made for the presence of aneurisms.

REMOVAL OF THORACIC ORGANS.

The heart. Except under special circumstances, it is convenient at this stage of the post-mortem examination to remove the heart from the body, and this is best done by grasping it in the left hand by the ventricles, drawing the heart gently upwards so that the great veins may be seen on the ventral aspect (Pl. IV fig. 7), and then, with the knife held at right angles to these veins, the inferior vena cava, the left and right pulmonary veins, the superior vena cava, the pulmonary artery and the aorta are in turn divided. After the inferior vena cava is divided the heart is so freed that an incision through the remainder of the vessels close to their apparent attachment is not likely to injure any important structures. The heart should always be pulled upwards with great care, otherwise artificial injuries may be produced and these may lead to erroneous conclusions. Not uncommonly, with rough handling, the inner coat of the aorta, close to the heart, may be damaged.

The lungs. Any adhesions having now been broken down, the left lung is raised from the thoracic cavity, pulled forwards to the middle line with the left hand, and the vessels and other structures at the root divided from behind. The right lung is dealt with in a similar fashion.

The aorta is now more carefully examined for any sign of aneurism, and then it should be removed, together with the œsophagus, thoracic duct, and the tissues in the superior mediastinum and the neck.

If the post-mortem examination is an unrestricted one it is always advisable at this stage to remove the tongue, the pharyngeal and laryngeal structures along with the trachea, œsophagus, aorta, etc.

For this purpose the skin of the neck is reflected from the anterior and lateral surfaces so that the muscles forming the floor of the mouth are completely exposed. By under cutting, the skin incision need not extend right to the tip of the chin, and this shortening of the incision is always advisable, as otherwise when the body is dressed the extreme end of the incision may be seen ; and the pathologist should always consider that the exposure of a wound, which to him may be a very trivial matter, may cause a considerable amount of trouble and annoyance to a sensitive relative or friend.

With a sharp scalpel or bistoury the structures forming the floor of the mouth are divided by incisions which, starting at the symphysis menti, pass backwards on each side close to the ramus of each half of the lower jaw. The tongue is pulled downwards through the incision, the soft palate is separated, and by careful dissection the pillars of the fauces, the tonsils, the pharyngeal muscles and the retro-pharyngeal tissues can be easily separated. Still exerting traction on the tongue and cutting where necessary close to the vertebra, there is practically no difficulty in removing, with the tissues already partially separated, the glands at the angle of the jaws, the upper cervical glands, the sublingual and submaxillary glands, the structures in the carotid sheath, the thoracic duct, the œsophagus, the trachea, larynx, the thyroid and thymus glands, and the aorta—in fact all the important structures from the tongue to the upper surface of the diaphragm.

Modifications of procedure. I have described what I believe to be the most satisfactory routine method for the removal of the thoracic organs, but necessarily the pathologist will have to vary this method when dealing with different cases, and it does not seem to me that it would be profitable to discuss all the modifications in procedure which might arise in any given case. The pathologist will naturally decide what method will best serve his purpose in any particular case. There are however a few points which seem worthy of mention.

In cases of pericarditis, where there are adhesions either recent or of old standing, it is well to remove the pericardium with the heart, the pulmonary vessels and the aorta being cut outside the sac and in cases of aneurismal dilatation of the aorta or where the history of the case points to the possibility of thrombosis or embolism in the pulmonary vessels, it is better to remove the whole of the thoracic viscera *en bloc.* The cervical structures are dissected off the vertebræ in the manner already described, and by pulling on these structures the thoracic viscera are very easily removed, if adhesions in the pleural sac have already been dealt with. The œsophagus is cut close to the diaphragm, after having previously been ligatured below the diaphragm. This latter precaution is necessary to avoid the contents of the stomach getting into the thoracic cavity.

Having removed all the organs from the thorax a careful examination is made of the ribs, the vertebræ and the costal pleura for the presence of fractures, tuberculosis, new growths, etc.

The Abdominal Contents.

The relative positions of the organs should be ascertained before any disturbance of the parts takes place, and note made of alterations in position.

Liver. In the right mammary line in a healthy adult the liver extends up to the level of the lower border of the fifth rib and, in the middle line, to that of the sixth chondro-sternal articulation. The lower border crosses the middle line almost midway between the tip of the ensiform cartilage and the umbilicus. The fundus of the gall bladder is seen near the angle between the outer edge of the rectus and the costal margin.

Displacements of the liver. Congenital transposition is uncommon but acquired displacements are frequent. The most common form is a downward displacement with a rotation on the antero-posterior axis—the right lobe may be considerably below its normal level. Note should be made of these displacements and the cause sought. The most usual causes are increase in the volume of the thoracic contents, or pressure on the lower ribs from without.

Stomach. When the stomach is empty the pylorus lies in the middle line or a little to the right of the mesial plane. The greater curvature crosses the middle line about a finger's breadth above the umbilicus, or about half-way between the inferior border of the liver and the umbilicus.

Spleen. The spleen is placed obliquely and reaches from the level of the ninth thoracic spine to the first lumbar spine. A line drawn from the left sterno-clavicular joint to the tip of the eleventh rib bounds the anterior margin of the organ.

Displacement of the spleen. Congenital transposition associated with transposition of the other abdominal organs sometimes occurs. Slight displacements upwards or downwards may occur but are of comparatively little importance. If the displacement is well marked, the position of the spleen should be specially noted.

The kidneys lie on the last thoracic and two upper lumbar vertebræ, the right lying about one-third to half-an-inch lower than the left.

Displacements of the kidney. These are generally associated with a lax or abnormal mesentery (floating or movable kidney), but sometimes the kidney may become freely movable over a limited area on account of the absorption of the fatty bed in which it lies, or from a loosening of its connections consequent on pregnancy. All such displacements are recorded, and the exact position defined before the kidneys are removed from the body.

Examination should now be made for the presence of fluid, either in localised pockets or distributed generally in the peritoneal sac, for recent deposits of lymph, for recent or old standing adhesions between the various coils of the intestine, or between the intestine and the other abdominal viscera. The mesenteric glands and those in the hilus of the liver and at the lesser curvature of the stomach should be investigated, particularly with the object of determining the presence of caseation or of calcification. The region of the appendix should always be examined for the presence of adhesions, for signs of recent inflammation or for actual suppuration. The presence of tumours of the stomach, intestine, liver, etc. are looked for, and the finding of these may determine the method of removal of the organs, *e.g.* cancerous nodules in the liver will at once suggest that the stomach and the liver should not be separated before removal from the body, or again a cancerous mass at the pyloric region will again distinctly indicate removal of the stomach, the duodenum and the liver together. Where fluid is present in the peritoneal cavity, portions of it should be removed into sterile test tubes for histological and bacteriological examination.

In certain cases, the character of the fluid found in the peritoneal sac will suggest to the pathologist a special line of examination. Thus, *hæmorrhage* in the cavity will call for special examination for a ruptured aortic aneurism, a rupture of one of the organs, *e.g.* the liver, intense inflammatory reaction, fracture of the pelvis, injury of the bladder, rupture of a tubal pregnancy, rupture of a degenerated vessel, etc. The main mass of the blood may be found either in the peritoneal sac or in the retro-peritoneal tissues. Where *suppuration* has occurred, pus may be found anterior to the peritoneal sac, in it, or retroperitoneally. When lying on the surface only, it may be secondary to wounds in the abdominal wall, but when the peritoneal sac contains pus the stomach, the duodenum and the intestines should be specially examined for ulceration and perforation, and the region of the appendix should be carefully looked at. When the purulent exudate is behind the peritoneum it may be caused by or associated with suppuration in or around the kidney, in the iliac bone, in the sacro-iliac joint, in the psoas or in the cæcal region. Subdiaphragmatic collections of pus can usually be traced to the region of the cæcum or the appendix. In cases of *ascites* unless some cause for the accumulation of serous fluid in the peritoneal sac is found from the clinical history of the case or from obvious pathological conditions, *e.g.* chronic heart disease, cirrhosis of the liver, chronic Bright's disease, tuberculosis or cancer of the peritoneum, it is desirable before the removal of any of the viscera to examine carefully for tumours which may press upon and obstruct the portal vessels or the thoracic duct. If the fluid is chylous, special investigation of the thoracic duct and its radicles should be made for rupture or for obstruction by tumours, by enlarged (tuberculous) glands, or by chronic inflammatory changes in or around the duct. In *acute inflammatory* conditions the fluid may not be abundant but its character is always distinctive.

It is richly albuminous, and fibrin is found deposited over the tissues in greater or less amount. In such cases careful examination should be made of the stomach and duodenum, as far as they can at this stage be exposed, for the presence of ruptured ulcers. The intestine and particularly the appendix should also be examined for ulceration or necrotic conditions. The coils of the intestine may be merely glued together by recent lymph or they may be firmly adherent by fibrous tissue— the result of old-standing inflammation of a simple or of a tuberculous nature. The positions of these *adhesions* should be noted, and special attention given as to whether they are causing actual constriction of the bowel.

It is very common to find adhesions in the region of the appendix, and between the cæcum, the hepatic and splenic flexures, and the abdominal parietes or the abdominal organs. Wilkie has pointed out that adhesions, some of which are congenital in origin (Jackson's membrane), are frequently found in the cæco-colic region, giving rise to definite cæcal stasis. Adhesions between the liver, spleen and diaphragm or the abdominal parietes are comparatively common. In all the areas in which adhesions are present, the pathologist should examine for any evidence of tuberculosis or of malignant disease. Tuberculosis may shew itself in the form of small miliary granulations scattered over both visceral and parietal layers of the peritoneum, as larger nodules with distinct contraction and thickening of the omentum, or merely by enlargement and caseation or calcification of the mesenteric glands.

Malignant disease may present definite isolated tumours varying much in size, or small irregular pearl-like nodules scattered over both visceral and parietal peritoneum. Besides the secondary malignant tumours which may be found in any part of the abdomen and which may bring about matting together of the various organs and consequently cause difficulties in their removal, other conditions may be found which may necessitate an alteration in the method of performing the examination. There may be considerable destruction of the tissues, *e.g.* by extensive tuberculous ulceration in the intestine, or by colloid cancer. I have seen cases where the abdomen was almost completely filled with a jelly-like (colloid) material associated with extensive malignant and necrotic changes. Hydatid cysts may be found scattered all over the peritoneum and, in one case which I saw, so extensive was the infiltration, that it was difficult to differentiate the organs.

The appendix should be examined for any evidence of inflammation, and the hernial regions for any abnormality. The contents of hernial sacs should, if possible, be delivered and carefully examined for signs of inflammation or gangrene. In cases where the clinical history points to obstruction, very careful manipulation should take place in the search for the cause, lest the obstructing agent be torn or the obstruction reduced.

If intussusception is present, the intussuscepted part, together with several inches of the bowel above, and if possible below, should be removed, hardened in preserving fluid and, later, sections should be made in order to determine the exact condition which was present.

REMOVAL OF THE ABDOMINAL ORGANS.

Having made this general examination of the abdomen, the viscera should now be removed in the following order :

(1) Small intestine. (2) Spleen. (3) Large intestine. (4) Liver, stomach, duodenum and pancreas. (5) Kidneys and suprarenals. (6) Pelvic organs.

1. *Small intestine.* The mesenteric attachment should be separated close to the intestine. After a preliminary incision of 3 or 4 inches has been made through the mesentery close to the bowel at the most convenient place, the separation is best continued by holding the bowel in the left hand so as to straighten out the mesentery, and then with a very sharp knife cutting the mesentery at right angles to the stretched bowel (Pl. IV fig. 8). The separation should be continued upwards to the duodenum, and downwards to within six inches of the ileo-cæcal valve. The bowel should then be double ligatured at each end;

Plate IV

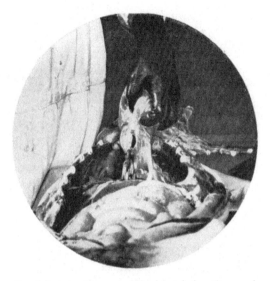

Fig. 7. Shewing the pulling up of the heart before the vessels are cut.

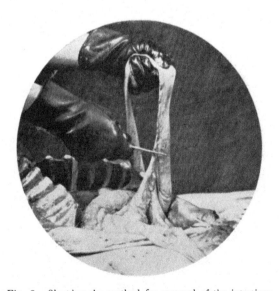

Fig. 8. Shewing the method for removal of the intestines.

and removed by cutting between the ligatures. By this method the bowel can be removed very rapidly, with practically no risk of damage, and when removed it should be possible to straighten it completely, without leaving irregular folds or bends.

2. *Spleen.* If there are no adhesions the spleen is pulled up from its bed with the left hand, and its attachments (vessels, etc.) cut through at the hilus. In dealing with acute poisonings (toxic or other) the spleen is usually very soft, and unless great care is taken in handling it, laceration is almost certain to take place. Where there are adhesions, these must be separated carefully before the spleen can be pulled forward.

In cases where the spleen is much enlarged, *e.g.* in medullary leukæmia, it is advisable to remove it before dealing with the intestines.

3. *Large intestine.* Commencing at the cæcal region the large intestine is usually easily separated by a few incisions through the loose tissue connecting it to the abdominal wall. The transverse colon must be carefully separated from the duodenum and the stomach. The descending colon should be separated as far down as the brim of the pelvis, where a double ligature should be applied and the bowel cut between the ligatures. The rectum is best removed with the pelvic organs. In removing the large intestine care should be taken not to cut into the ureters.

4. *Liver, stomach, duodenum and pancreas.* In many cases it is very desirable that these organs should be removed *en masse*, in order that a careful examination should be made of the bile and pancreatic ducts throughout their course. This removal is best accomplished by dissecting from below upwards, separating the duodenum, the pancreas, the liver and the stomach, and finally dividing the diaphragm on each side from its lateral attachments and removing it with the organs. Care should be taken to avoid injury of the right suprarenal capsule in dissecting up the right lobe of the liver, and too much pressure should not be exerted, lest rupture of ulcers in the stomach or the duodenum take place.

In many cases the liver is removed alone before the stomach, duodenum and pancreas. This operation I find most conveniently done in the following manner:

(a) Raise the right lobe of the liver slightly and, with the fingers, separate the right suprarenal capsule from it.

(b) Pass a cartilage knife or a bistoury backwards and outwards between the diaphragm and the upper surface of the right lobe of the liver, the handle of the knife lying close to the suspensory ligament. With the point of the knife puncture the diaphragm at its posterior attachment and cut upwards and inwards so as to completely separate the right half of the diaphragm from the liver.

(c) With the left hand raise the left lobe of the liver and cut through the attachments towards the vertebral column.

(d) With the hand the right lobe is separated from the areolar tissue on its posterior aspect.

(e) The suspensory ligament is cut through.

(f) Little difficulty will now be experienced in raising the liver from its bed and giving free access to the bile ducts and vessels in the hilus. Pulling the liver to the right with the left hand, the vessels, etc. at the hilus are cut through and the organ is thus completely removed from the body.

The stomach, duodenum and pancreas may now be removed by careful dissection from below or from above, care being taken in the manipulation lest ulcers in the stomach or in the duodenum be artificially ruptured.

5. *The kidneys and suprarenals.* An incision is made through the peritoneum at the anterior aspect of the kidney, and, passing the hand through this opening, the kidney and its suprarenal capsule can be separated from the surrounding tissues and freed to such an extent that they are attached by the ureter and vessels only. The ureter can be dissected as far as the brim of the pelvis, or in special cases right to the bladder. Ordinarily however the vessels and the ureter are cut near the kidney and the organ thus removed.

6. *The pelvic organs.* If the peritoneum is cut through round the brim of the pelvis the hand can be introduced and the contents of the pelvis easily separated, except at the anterior

surface where they are attached to the external organs of generation. This anterior attachment is cut through as close as possible to the bone. Then the rectum is cut through close to the anus, and, in the female, the vagina close to the labia. Care should be taken to avoid cutting the external skin in these parts. In the male, the contents will comprise the rectum, the bladder with the remaining parts of the ureters and the prostate ; in the female, in addition to the rectum and bladder will be found the uterus, with its tubes, the ovaries and the upper part of the vagina.

7. *The solar plexus*, the *receptaculum chyli*, the *aorta*, the *inferior vena cava* and its tributaries, the *hæmolymph* and other *glands* can now be examined *in situ* and portions removed if more detailed examination is deemed necessary.

The bones of the pelvis and the vertebral column are examined for any sign of fracture, of necrosis, of deformity or of tumour formation, and careful note made of the situation, the extent and the character of any such condition which may be found.

The methods which have been described are applicable to the majority of cases, but the intelligence of the pathologist must be his guide in cases which present special features. Thus in cases of extensive peritoneal adhesions it will be obvious that the intestines cannot be examined by the ordinary routine method. The whole of the abdominal organs should be removed *en masse*, and the various organs dissected from this mass in the most suitable way. Again, large tumours in the abdomen which have formed adhesions require special treatment, and in such cases it may be found necessary to remove portions of the intestine at irregular intervals in the length of the bowel.

CHAPTER IV

EXAMINATION OF THE THORACIC CONTENTS

If the whole of the cervical tissues have been removed with the thoracic contents, any gross changes should be noted, and the mass placed with the dorsal surface uppermost. The œsophagus and the pharynx should be slit open from below upwards and in the mesial line posteriorly, and then the trachea and larynx opened in a similar manner—the incision being carried well into the larger bronchi. An examination of these structures should now be made, but a description of the method to be followed will be more conveniently given later (p. 91).

If necessary, the thoracic duct can at this stage be dissected out, the aorta opened from below upwards and any pathological condition in the aorta, e.g. aneurism, or in the posterior mediastinal tissues, e.g. sarcoma, accurately described.

In cases where death from pulmonary embolism or pulmonary thrombosis is suspected, the extra-pulmonary vessels should be opened very carefully and the incision continued into the intra-pulmonary branches and tributaries in order to search for the suspected embolus or thrombus.

The lungs are now separated from the heart by cutting through the pulmonary vessels and the bronchi on each side, as close as possible to the root of the lung, and then after opening the pericardium, if this has not already been done, the heart is separated by cutting through the great vessels close to their exit from, or entrance into, the pericardial sac. If the pericardium is adherent to the epicardium, the great vessels are divided just outside the sac and thus the heart with its coverings is separated from the remaining mediastinal tissues.

THE PERICARDIUM AND HEART.

The pericardium. The main changes in the pericardium have already been referred to in the examination preliminary to removal of the organs. At this stage therefore there is little further to be done except to examine more in detail the extent and the character of any inflammatory exudate, the cause of any hæmorrhagic effusion, and to determine the extent and character of any adhesions which may be present, or the degree to which the pericardium may have become infiltrated by tuberculosis or by new growths—such as lympho-sarcoma or, less commonly, cancer.

The heart. Careful examination must be made of the epicardium, attention being specially directed to the presence and the extent of any fibrinous exudate, indicating acute pericarditis. This exudate may be very slight in amount and may be found only in the region of the bases of the great vessels, about the auriculo-ventricular groove. When quite recent, the exudate strips off readily, leaving a smooth glistening surface. Very soon it becomes vascularised and then cannot be stripped so easily.

In cases of tuberculosis, the exudate is usually much thicker than in the non-tuberculous cases, and is definitely adherent to the epicardium.

In septicæmia, and in poisoning from various causes, petechial hæmorrhages are very common on the surface of the epicardium, particularly, in my experience, near the base of the heart and on its posterior aspect.

Any excess of fatty deposit, especially over the right ventricle, should be noted, and also the presence of thickened patches of the epicardium—the so-called milk spots. The exact site and extent of these should be recorded.

Other pathological conditions such as infarction—*myo-malacia cordis*, primary or secondary malignant growths, syphilitic gummata, etc. should be described, as far as is possible, before the cavities are opened. The condition of the coronary arteries as seen from the external surface, such as tortuosity and dilatation—local or general—should also be noted. The general shape and size of the heart should be recorded, with special reference to atrophy and to hypertrophy of the heart as a whole, and of its individual chambers.

Method of examining the heart after removal from the peri-cardial sac. It is advisable to adopt a systematic method of examining the individual chambers of the heart and I have found it convenient to commence with the right auricle and follow the direction of the blood-flow.

Right auricle. Any evidence of dilatation of the auricle or its appendix is noted, and then a curved, probe-pointed bistoury is passed from the inferior to the superior vena cava and the wall between these orifices cut through. From the centre of this incision a second cut is made obliquely into the beginning of the auricular appendix. The chamber is thus laid completely open. The blood clot with which it is frequently filled is carefully tilted out, a note being particularly made of the character of the clot in the auricular appendix and whether this is in direct connection with the clot in the auricle. It is frequently found that the clot in the appendix is firm and actually adherent to the wall. The clot having been removed, the tricuspid orifice should be carefully examined for the presence of vegetations, and, if these are present, portions of them should be removed at once and put into a sterile vessel or inoculated into a tube of broth or agar.

Before further examination of the auricle is made, the *right ventricle* should be opened. This is best done with a sharp-pointed bistoury which is plunged through the muscular wall at the anterior aspect of the ventricle about midway between the apex and base of the chamber at a distance of $\frac{1}{2}$ to $\frac{3}{4}$ inch ($1\frac{1}{2}$ to 2 cm.) to the right of the septum ventriculorum. The incision is continued downwards to the apex and upwards towards the base of the heart, but at first not extending up to the commencement of the pulmonary artery (Pl. V). A general examination of the interior of the cavity can be made through this opening, and any clots displaced. By a little intelligent manipulation the flaps of the tricuspid valve may be seen, and any evidence of recent endocarditis, which has escaped observation from the auricular aspect, noted. By cutting the pulmonary artery short, and holding the heart with the apex resting in the palm of the left hand, the cusps of the pulmonary valves may be seen and any evidence of vegetations on them detected. It is important to make this observation before any water is run through the pulmonary orifice, so that

Plate V

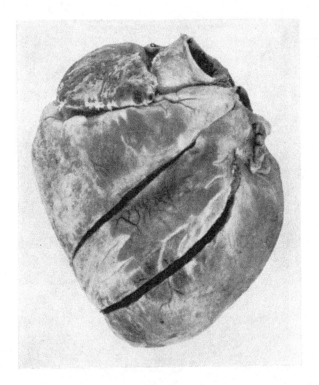

Fig. 9. Shewing incisions for opening the right
and left ventricles.

bacteriological examination may be undertaken with as little risk of contamination as possible. Before the cusps can be seen it is often necessary to detach clots, and the character of these and their place of attachment should always be observed.

If no vegetations are found, and bacteriological examination is not deemed necessary, the heart is again held with the apex in the palm of the left hand and water is allowed to run into the pulmonary artery to test the extent of closure of the orifice by the cusps of the valves. When completely competent, no water should flow through the artery into the ventricle. In testing this competency of the valves it is important to make quite sure that there is no clot lying between the cusps and preventing their complete closure.

The circumferential measurement of the opening of the orifice may now be taken with cones if the pathologist deems this desirable. (Shennan gives this measurement as normally 8·5 to 9·1 cm.)

A curved, probe-pointed bistoury is now passed from the ventricular opening through the pulmonary artery and an incision made between the two anterior cusps. The right ventricle is in this way completely opened.

Left auricle. A probe-pointed bistoury is passed from one of the *right* pulmonary veins through the left lower pulmonary vein and an incision made in this line through the wall of the auricle, and this incision is continued into the left auricular appendix. The cavity is in this way completely opened up. Blood clots are carefully removed, note being made, as on the right side as to their character, etc. The mitral orifice should now be examined for vegetations, and if these are present small portions should be removed for bacteriological examination.

Left ventricle. This should be opened from the anterior aspect by an incision made in the same manner as, and parallel with, that for the opening of the right ventricle (Pl. V fig. 9). Through this opening clots are carefully removed from the chamber, and the mitral segments are more thoroughly examined for vegetations. Having as far as possible satisfied oneself that there are no vegetations requiring bacteriological examination, the forefinger is passed into the mitral orifice from above to detect any evidence of stenosis, of chronic endocarditis or other pathological change. The circumference of the orifice may be taken (normally 9·7 to 11·1 cm.—Shennan).

Before further examination of this chamber is made, the aortic orifice is carefully examined. This may be done merely by cutting the aorta short, holding the heart with the apex in the palm of the left hand and looking into the aorta ; but a much more satisfactory inspection can be made without damage to the valves, or to vegetations which may be present, by the following procedure which was first demonstrated to me by my former colleague, Professor D. A. Welsh, of the University of Sydney.

The aorta being cut short a probe-pointed bistoury is passed down the inner surface of the aorta into the right coronary artery, and this vessel, along with the aorta above it, is slit open. In a similar manner the bistoury is passed into the left coronary artery and a like incision made. These incisions open up the aorta so thoroughly that the cusps are distinctly seen, and most pathological conditions of them can be accurately observed.

This method is specially valuable in cases of vegetative endocarditis, where a bacteriological examination is required, as full exposure of the vegetations is made with practically no risk of contamination. It also has the advantage of ensuring that the coronary arteries will be opened up and examined—a matter of importance and one which is very often omitted.

If no vegetations are present, or if sufficient material has been removed for bacteriological examination, the aortic segments may be palpated, and the size of the orifice determined either with the finger or with the measuring cone (the circumference is given by Shennan as normally 7·3 to 8·2 cm.). If it is desired to test the competence of the valves by the water test, this is best done before the coronary arteries and the aorta have been slit up, but if there are vegetations present, or if a sufficient view cannot be obtained in order to determine this, the water test should be omitted. In order that the left ventricle may be further opened up, a bistoury is passed from the opening already made in the ventricular wall through the aortic orifice and between the two most suitable cusps, and the incision made from within outwards through the muscular wall. In making this incision care should be taken to avoid, as far as possible, injury to the pulmonary artery and to the mitral valve. If a more minute examination is required of the auricular aspects of the mitral valve than can be obtained by the method described, the bistoury is passed through the mitral orifice in a line passing obliquely outwards from the inner side of the larger papillary muscle to the outer angle of the orifice, and the muscular wall between the edge of the bistoury and the outer aspect of the ventricle cut through. Thus the mitral orifice is completely opened and the valve segments can be thoroughly examined.

Before proceeding to the examination of the opened heart the coronary arteries should be more completely slit up with a fine probe-pointed bistoury or fine probe-pointed scissors.

Examination is now made of the various chambers for evidences of hypertrophy, dilatation, atrophy, and for the presence of blood clots entangled in the columnæ carnæ; the colour and friability of the muscle, as indicating brown atrophy or fatty degeneration; the condition of the endocardium, with special reference to thickening, opacity, petechial hæmorrhages, etc.; and the condition of the valves as to acute or chronic endocarditis, destructive changes, contraction and retraction, chronic fibrous thickening, fenestration, congenital abnormalities, etc.

The circumferential measurement of the tricuspid orifice may be taken at this point (normally 12·9 to 13·7 cm.—Shennan).

The dilatation of the chambers is shewn, not only by their large size, but also by the flattening of the muscular bundles, the hypertrophy of the wall by the increased thickness and more marked firmness of the muscle, and the atrophy by the thinning of the wall, the reduction in size of the cavity and the dark brown colour of the muscle—" brown atrophy."

The measurements of the length of the cavities and the

thickness of the walls of the ventricles should be ascertained.

Normally the right ventricle in the adult measures 8 to 9 cm. in length, internally from the opening of the pulmonary artery to the apex of the ventricle, and the thickness of its walls varies from ·5 to ·7 cm., a short distance below the auriculoventricular groove, to ·3 cm., close to the apex.

The left ventricle has an internal measurement about equal to that of the right, but the thickness of the walls is greater, varying from 1 to 1·5 cm., opposite the base of the anterior papillary muscle, to 0·5 cm. at the apex.

The wall of the left auricle usually measures 2 to 3 mm., that of the right being slightly less.

The presence of blood clots should be ascertained and their character noted—the ante-mortem clots being pale and firm and either attached to the endocardium or lying free in some of the chambers (" ball thrombi "), and the post-mortem ones being dark and friable or pale and friable in those cases in which they are composed mainly of serum from which the red blood corpuscles have been separated.

The appearance of the muscular wall is of great importance. Normally it is firm and of a reddish colour. It may become extremely friable as in fatty degeneration or in necrotic changes which may follow obstruction to the coronary arteries—*myomalacia cordis*—or it may become more firm and resistant in cases of hypertrophy or where there has been an overgrowth of fibrous tissue—a condition which may result from myocarditis or merely from a deficient blood supply brought about by degenerative changes in the arteries. The brown colouration in " brown atrophy " has already been noted. The infiltration of the muscle by fat in cases of adiposity is usually easily observed, and is specially seen towards the apex of the right ventricle.

Fatty degeneration, which gives a yellowish colour to the muscle when it is diffuse, is often patchy in distribution and then is best observed as pale areas in the papillary muscles or in the muscles lying immediately under the endocardium in the left ventricle—"the thrush-breast " or " tabby cat " appearance.

The white fibrous bands of interstitial myocarditis may sometimes be seen, but not uncommonly this condition is detected only after microscopical examination. Thickening with opacity of the endocardium usually results from prolonged irritation in the cavity—such as accompanies stenosis of the valve segments. Thus in mitral stenosis the endocardium of the left auricle may become greatly thickened. This condition however is not in itself of any special importance. Petechial hæmorrhages are sometimes seen under the endocardium and their position should be noted. A careful examination of all the valve segments and cusps should now be made and special notes made of the position and extent of any chronic fibrous changes, of calcification, of contraction or retraction, of rupture and of any abnormalities. Where there are vegetations present, their exact site and extent, and their general characters should be recorded. Careful examination should be made for destructive changes of and for aneurisms in the valves. The aneurisms are often very small and may be concealed among the vegetations, and their orifices are therefore sometimes found with difficulty. They usually bulge towards the ventricle when situated on the aortic valves and towards the auricle when on the mitral segments.

Careful examination should be made of stenosed orifices to determine the cause and the degree of the stenosis, whether there is calcification present, and, in the mitral and tricuspid segments, whether the chordæ tendineæ have been ruptured or are thickened, shortened or adherent to one another. The papillary muscles should be examined for fibrosis. The mitral orifice is said to admit, in its normal condition, two fingers and the tricuspid three. This is necessarily an extremely rough and inaccurate measurement, but it is often of value in determining whether the orifice is grossly narrowed or dilated.

The coronary arteries should be examined for atheromatous changes and the site of the change noted—very commonly the openings into the aorta shew the change in a marked degree while the rest of the vessel is comparatively healthy. In cases of infarction in the heart, the vessels should be searched for a thrombus or an embolus.

Congenital abnormalities are often overlooked. The most important is a patent foramen ovale which is often valved and therefore may not give evidence of its presence during life. The fossa ovalis in the auricular septum should in every case be examined for this condition. Sometimes the opening is so marked that it may occupy the whole area of the fossa. Not at all uncommonly this defect is associated with patency of the ductus arteriosus and narrowing of the pulmonary artery.

Defects in the auricular septum are not common. There may be entire absence of the septum or there may be merely an opening between the two ventricles limited to the *pars membranacea*.

It is not uncommon to find defects in the valve segments—the aortic orifice may shew two or four cusps and the tricuspid four. More commonly stenosis, which must be regarded as congenital, may be found at the pulmonary valve or at the tricuspid orifice. These conditions are generally associated with other congenital abnormalities. Certain abnormalities in the number or in the arrangement of the great vessels may be found, but these are not of special pathological importance, though from the developmental standpoint they are of interest, and should therefore be accurately described.

Weight of the heart. After the examination of the heart is completed it should be weighed—the average weight of the female heart is from 220 to 350 gm. and of the male 315 to 390 gm. The size of the individual must be considered before deciding that the heart is heavier or lighter than normal.

Microscopical examination. Small portions should now be cut from various parts of the heart and put in fixative for later histological examination. It is well to take sections from the wall of each ventricle and from the septum in every case, but special diseases will indicate to the pathologist the site from which the pieces should be removed, *e.g.* in cases of heart block it is desirable to examine the auriculo-ventricular bundle and other portions of the primitive muscular tissue of the heart, and for this purpose Ritchie[1] recommends that three

---

[1] Quoted by Shennan.

portions of tissue should be removed for examination by serial sections.

" (1) That portion of the wall of the right auricle and of the superior vena cava lying between the latter and the right auricular appendix.

(2) That portion of the cardiac septum extending backwards to the mouth of the coronary sinus and forwards so as to include the pars membranacea septi and the attachment of the septal cusp of the tricuspid valve.

(3) A portion of the ventricular wall close above the base of the anterior papillary muscle of the left ventricle."

In the first of these blocks will be found any pathological condition affecting the sino-auricular node, in the second, affections of the auriculo-ventricular node, the auriculo-ventricular bundle and its two main branches, and in the third any involvement of the Purkinje fibres. Again, in cases of rheumatism, Aschoff and Tawara and Carey Coombs have described specific nodules in the heart muscle and, for the careful examination of these, blocks of tissue should be cut from various regions.

Coombs writes as follows :

" (a) The nodules are very often immediately related to arteries. They appear to arise usually from the periarterial connective tissue, but sometimes from the tunica adventitia of the artery itself.

(b) Nodules are found in numbers, just under both serous layers, especially in the sub-pericardial tissues ; but they are most thickly sown in the central path of the myocardium. Sections of auricular walls have so far disclosed almost no nodules except under the endocardium close to the auriculo-ventricular ring.

(c) In the right ventricle they are scanty. The most productive sections were from a block of tissue close to the apex ; next to this came that portion of muscle bordering on the fibrous ring giving origin to the tricuspid flaps.

(d) The interventricular septum contains but few nodules.

(e) The wall of the left ventricle contains the bulk of the nodules. The nodules were sown most thickly at the origin of the aorta, at the apex close to the septum, and at the insertion of the ventricular wall into the fibrous ring of the mitral valve. They have also been found in the valves and in the chordæ tendineæ."

Thrombi in the heart.

Ante-mortem thrombi of two types may be found.

(1) Those which are attached to the wall by more or less firm adhesions. These are seen in the auricular appendices and frequently project for some distance into the auricle or they may be seen between the musculi pectinati in the auricles or entangled between the columnæ carnæ in the ventricles. These thrombi are pale or greyish in colour, firm, usually polypoid and, as has been already said, more or less adherent to the wall.

(2) Those which lie close in the cavities—the "ball thrombi." They are globular, fairly firm and are composed of laminated thrombus. They are most commonly found in the left auricle but may be seen in other cavities. They are comparatively uncommon.

Post-mortem clots are also of two types.

(1) The common dark clots which are found almost constantly in the various chambers and also in the vessels. They are not adherent to the walls, and merely consist of coagulated blood. Sometimes these clots are pale as in cases of leucocythæmia, or they may be of a yellowish colour. Not uncommonly we find pale yellowish clots lying on top of dark ones. This is merely due to the fact that the serum has become partially separated from the corpuscles and that it has formed a separate clot.

Whether pale or dark these clots are very friable and not adherent, though they may be entangled in the muscular bundles, and may thus appear as if they were actually adherent to the muscular wall.

(2) Firm, stringy, pale yellow clots are frequently found in the right side of the heart, especially in such diseases as lobar pneumonia. If carefully traced, it will usually be found that they commence in a mass of clot entangled in the muscular

bundles behind the auriculo-ventricular valve or in the columnæ near the apex. They extend upwards through the pulmonary artery and may form a cast of this vessel and its branches. Not uncommonly the clot may be traced backwards through the tricuspid orifice to the right auricle and the right auricular appendix. The distal end is usually dark in colour and friable. These clots can always be easily separated and, though more firmly attached to the heart than the first type of post-mortem clots, they are not truly adherent and organisation of them does not take place.

Similar, though usually less extensive, clots are sometimes found in the left side of the heart. The clots are usually called " agony " or " agonal " thrombi but they are not formed by blood plate separation as are the true thrombi ; and as they appear just at the end of life when the circulation is really failing, I have classed them with the post-mortem clots rather than with the ante-mortem thrombi.

The aorta and great vessels. These should be carefully opened up if this has not already been done and note particularly made of the condition of the inner coat. The most common pathological condition is atheroma. The position of the atheromatous patches, whether widely distributed or confined to the origin of the smaller vessels, the stage of development of the process—whether the very early raised pale areas or the advanced calcified areas—should be carefully described. Any evidence of dilatation should be sought, and, if there are definitely formed aneurisms present, these should be accurately described as to their size, their position, their shape and their contents, and any pathological conditions to which they may have given rise by pressure, such as erosion of bone, ulceration of soft structures, displacement of organs or tissues, etc. should be noted. Where the aneurism has ruptured, the site of the rupture must be sought. If dissecting aneurisms are present, the position of the blood and the extent to which it has invaded the walls must be noted.

The Lungs and the Respiratory Passages.

The lungs. Note has already been made in the preliminary examination of the pleural cavities, of adhesions, fluid, etc. The positions of the adhesions and their extent on the surface of the lung can be better appreciated now that the lungs have been removed from the thorax, and further details on these points should be given in the report.

The surfaces of both lungs are examined, special attention being directed to the following points :

(1) *Diffuse general or localised thickening*—the amount and the special site.

(2) The presence of greyish *tubercle granulations*, of larger nodules of *malignant disease*, of the pearly-looking, *fibrous nodules* so commonly associated with dust diseases, such as silicosis, care being taken to carefully distinguish between the fibrous nodules and the tubercle granulations.

(3) *Recent inflammatory changes*, evidenced by the presence of more or less fibrinous exudate. The site of this and its extent should receive special attention, and the exudate should be examined to find out whether it strips readily (recent) or whether adhesions have formed between it and the surface of the lung.

(4) Any evidence of *cavity formation*. This may be shewn by localised thickening of the pleura, but it frequently happens that in removing the lung, where there are superficial cavities, the tissue becomes lacerated and the cavities opened up.

(5) The presence of *emphysema*, as evidenced by the pale colour and the bulbous character of the lung tissue. The positions in which this condition is most evident are noted and whether it affects the whole or only part of the lung.

(6) *Collapse* of the lung is indicated in external examination by the firmness of the tissue, by its dark plum colour and frequently by the thickened pleura over the site. Small lobular areas of collapse are very common—and shew as dark areas depressed below the surface. The exact extent and the site of the collapsed areas are of importance in any report.

(7) *Infarcts.* These are generally found at the surface and are dark and hæmorrhagic in appearance, distinctly raised above the surface, and firm in consistence. These will be examined more in detail after the lungs have been incised.

(8) *Scars or cicatrices.* These are common at the apex and should always be looked for ; very often they are associated with firm fibrous tissue or with calcareous deposit (possibly in many cases they are healed foci of tuberculosis). Scarring may also be found in other parts in association with interstitial changes in the lung substance.

(9) Alteration in *size* of the lungs. The lungs may be increased or diminished in size in emphysema. They are usually increased in diseases which give rise to consolidation such as pneumonia and tuberculosis. These conditions are usually easily detected by external examination alone.

(10) The presence of *air* in the interstitial framework of the lung can generally be detected on examination of the surface (interstitial emphysema).

The weight of the lungs should now be taken. Shennan gives the following weights for a series of, presumably normal, lungs which he has examined.

Left lung. In females 1 lb. 3 oz. or 538 grammes and in males 1 lb. 10 oz. or 708 grammes.

Right lung. In females 1 lb. 4 oz. or 566 grammes and in males 1 lb. 12 oz. or 764 grammes.

These figures, he says, probably slightly overstate the normal weight of these organs.

The superficial examination having been completed, the bronchi and the vessels at the root of the lung should be investigated and the bronchial glands examined. Starting at the open end of the larger bronchi, and the larger vessels at the root of the lung, an incision is carried from this point into the lung substance, till a number of the smaller bronchi and vessels are opened up. By this method, clots or emboli are found, and any condition of degeneration of the walls of the vessels detected. The bronchi are examined for bronchitis, dilatation (bronchiectasis), accumulations of secretion, stenosis, and invasion by tumours, etc. In cases of bronchiectasis a very thorough examination of the bronchi should be made, and portions removed for histological examination. The secretion should be examined bacteriologically and it may be necessary to examine the bronchial mucous membrane for the presence of organisms. In such cases, it is important to select areas which have not been contaminated during the preliminary operation of opening up the bronchi. The clinical history of any case may give information to the pathologist which will lead him to take such special precautions in opening up the bronchial channels, or the pulmonary vessels as may be required when the presence of a small foreign body is suspected or where there has been sudden death from a supposed pulmonary embolism, and particularly in cases where special bacteriological examination is desirable, and I would therefore again urge that the pathologist should insist on the main facts of every case being supplied to him before he commences his examination.

In examining for bronchitis the essential points to be noted are the degree of œdema and congestion of the mucous membrane, its colour, and the amount and the character of the secretion. In the *acute* cases the congestion and œdema are marked, the secretion is in excess and may be thin or thick, mucous, muco-purulent or purulent ; in the *chronic* types the colour may be purplish or purplish-grey and the secretion is usually viscid and muco-purulent. There may be thickening or atrophy of the mucous membrane, which in many cases is also granular in appearance. In other cases a definite membrane may be present on the mucous surface—plastic bronchitis. Such membranes are composed largely of fibrin and should always be carefully examined for the presence of bacteria and particularly for *B. diphtheria*. Membranes of a similar nature are sometimes observed in cases of gangrenous or putrid bronchitis, and, in such cases, there is usually some degree of bronchiectasis. The bronchiectatic cavities are generally detected without difficulty and are often filled with very putrid secretion. Bacteriological examination of the secretion should always be made, and, especially because at later stages in the examination, pyæmic abscesses may be found in various parts of the body, *e.g.* in the brain, and these may have as their primary focus the septic changes in a bronchiectatic cavity, and therefore it may be of importance to determine that the causal organism is identical in the primary and in the secondary focus.

The lung itself is now incised and examined. The first incision should extend from apex to base and from the outer surface almost to the root of the lung. Two or more incisions should then be made more or less at right angles to the first incision and extending from it to the anterior edges of the various lobes. All these incisions should just fall short of passing through the whole thickness of the lung. Special incisions may be necessary in special cases, *e.g.* in localised areas of collapse, areas of broncho-pneumonia, suppurative foci, infarcts, etc., but in the majority of cases, it will be found that the incisions which have been made in the first instance enable most of the pathological conditions of the lung to be examined in a satisfactory manner. The incisions in the two lungs should, as far as possible, correspond with one another and, in making them, it is therefore convenient to follow a definite plan.

Right lung. This is placed with its posterior (dorsal) surface lying on the table and the root directed to the operator's right hand. It is grasped firmly with the left hand—the thumb being at the outer surface near the lower margin and the four fingers on the upper surface. An incision is made with a long-bladed knife from apex to base of the lung—the incision passing midway between the thumb and the fingers of the left hand of the operator and being directed from the outer aspect towards the root. In many cases this incision is sufficient to enable a satisfactory examination of the lung to be made, but it is sometimes advisable to make a second or even a third incision at right angles to the first one and passing outwards towards the anterior margin of the lung.

Left lung. This is placed in a similar position with however the root directed towards the left side of the operator. In grasping the lung the fingers will be on the outer aspect. The incisions will be similar in position and direction to those in the right lung.

In the examination of the cut surface of the lung the following points have to be observed :

A. *On inspection.* Normally the lung is of a pinkish colour, though very commonly the lower lobe is dark red on account of the presence of hypostatic congestion. In pneumonia the whole of the lung or of one lobe or of part of a lobe may be red (red hepatisation) or grey (grey hepatisation), but more commonly the grey is more marked and at the proximal parts of the solid area the grey may gradually shade off into a reddish tint—(the more recently affected part). The reddish-grey or greyish areas may be irregularly scattered throughout the lung tissue (broncho-pneumonia). In collapse the tissue is of a bluish-red or purplish colour, or sometimes, where there is much associated congestion, a darker slaty colour. In infarction the localised wedge- or often oval-shaped area, is of a very dark (hæmorrhagic) colour. In hypostatic pneumonia or in hypostatic congestion the lower lobe is dark red in colour, and in the lungs of coal miners the whole of the tissue is black from the accumulated coal-dust. The lung is paler than normal in case of anæmia and also in emphysema.

Localised alterations in colour are seen in the dark (almost black), pigmented, fibrous bands or nodules associated with interstitial overgrowth in tuberculosis and in dust-diseases. The carbon pigment collects especially in the peripheral parts of the newly formed fibrous tissue. These pigmented fibrous nodules are a very marked feature in the lungs of grinders, and particularly in those parts of the lung which have not become extensively involved by tuberculosis.

In some cases of syphilis the fibrous tissue is said to remain unpigmented. This " white pneumonia " is described by Schultz as occurring in non-syphilitic children dying within the first two or three months after birth. I have never seen a case presenting this syphilitic interstitial pneumonia in a young child, but certainly in adults the fibrous tissue in syphilitic cases becomes pigmented.

A granular appearance of the cut surface, due to escape of exudate from the air spaces, is common in lobar pneumonia.

The position, the size and the general characteristics of any cavities which may be present should be recorded. Special attention should be directed to the character of the walls of the cavity, to the vessels passing through it, to any evidence of aneurismal dilatation, and to the amount of fibrous tissue surrounding the cavity. Communicating channels between the cavity and bronchi should be looked for.

The presence of tumours, their position, size, consistence, colour, etc. should be noted, and various incisions may be necessary to determine these points accurately.

Hæmorrhage into the lung is of great importance and, where this has taken place, its source should be sought. It may arise from the rupture of an aneurism of the aorta which has been pressing upon the lung and which has eroded into a bronchus, or the rupture of an aneurism on a pulmonary vessel in a phthisical cavity. Small hæmorrhages occur in chronic venous congestion, in hypostasis, in infarction, in malignant disease and in some of the infective fevers. Pulmonary hæmorrhage is a characteristic feature of wool-sorter's disease (bronchial anthrax), and may occur in leucocythæmia, scurvy and hæmophilia. It is said also to result from the presence of such animal parasites as *Distoma pulmonale* and hydatids. Minute hæmorrhages have been described in phosphorus poisoning, chloroform poisoning, and in fat embolism, and I have seen similar hæmorrhages in very acute and rapidly fatal pneumococcic infections without definite consolidation.

Infarcts in the lung have been already referred to. Their regular shape and their consistence usually distinguish them quite readily from hæmorrhages. The causal embolus or thrombus should be sought in these cases.

B. *On palpation.* By passing the forefinger gently over the surface of the lung, solid areas such as those of broncho-pneumonia or the nodules of fibrosis which are produced by dust diseases are generally very easily recognised, and their limits can usually be defined. Firmer but gradually increasing pressure will differentiate the true consolidation of pneumonia from the solid lung of collapse or of chronic venous congestion. In pneumonia the tissue is very friable and breaks down under the pressure; in collapse the lung is firm and fleshy and pressure produces no laceration ; in chronic venous congestion and in œdema fluid is gradually pressed out of the tissue, but there is no laceration and the tissue feels firm and indurated.

In cases of simple œdema the lung is spongy and, on pressure, watery and frothy fluid exudes; in acute congestion the same spongy character is noted but the fluid is reddish (blood stained) ; in chronic venous congestion and in hypostatic conditions the spongy character is not so marked, because of the associated overgrowth of fibrous tissue or of collapse, and exuded fluid is of a brownish or dark reddish colour. This alteration in colour is particularly well seen in cases of chronic venous congestion. In anthracosis (coal-miner's lung) the fluid is of a dark greyish colour, but never quite black. In emphysema the lung is spongy but very dry and little or no blood can be pressed out of it. In suppurative and in gangrenous conditions pus and necrotic tissues can be pressed from the lung. Increase of fibrous tissue in any part of the lung, such as is seen in syphilitic and other forms of interstitial pneumonia, always produces an increase in the consistence and toughness of the lung. The apices should always be examined for firm fibrous or calcareous nodules and any area where scarring of the lung tissue has been observed should be examined for similar nodules. In my experience these scars are specially found in syphilitic cases in the lower lobes, and are associated with the presence of gummata, whereas in chronic tuberculous cases they are found at or near the apices.

In cases of tuberculosis, accurate descriptions of the distribution, the general characters, including the shape and the size of the areas, the presence of fibrosis and its distribution, the consistence of the nodules and the general characters of any cavities that may be present, should be given, and the examination of the bronchial glands is of special importance. The ragged irregular cavities or the irregular caseous areas which are usually raised above the surface and easily broken down, are characteristic of the more acute processes, while the cavities with smooth walls or the firmer irregular areas with a considerable amount of fibrous tissue in and around them are specially seen in the more chronic cases. It should always be remembered that the two conditions may be present in the same lung. In examining cases which present on inspection the appearance of wide-spread acute miliary tuberculosis, the consistence of the nodules should be noted, as the condition may be simulated by very minute purulent foci. In tuberculosis the nodules are comparatively firm whereas in the purulent cases they are soft and often slightly yellowish in colour. I have seen a case of general pulmonary streptothrix infection which was mistaken by several pathologists and clinicians for acute miliary tuberculosis. Nodules due to infection by B. *mallei* or B. *lepra* may occur in the lungs, but they are comparatively rare and the history of the case will prevent any error, and microscopical examination will clear up any difficulty in the diagnosis.

Hydatid cysts may occur in the lung, but these are not likely to lead to any confusion.

Of the tumours, sarcomata, endotheliomata and carcinomata may occur, but no pathologist of experience will omit a microscopical examination before giving a diagnosis of such cases.

Having now made a careful naked eye examination of the lung, portions should be removed and put in some fixing solution for histological examination. No matter what is the nature of the case, this should be a routine procedure, and the parts from which the blocks are taken must be determined according to the conditions which are found in the lung on naked eye examination.

CHAPTER V

EXAMINATION OF THE ABDOMINAL CONTENTS

EXAMINATION OF THE VARIOUS ORGANS.

This may be done in any order, but it is always advisable to follow a definite system and I suggest the following :

Liver, stomach, duodenum and pancreas. If the liver has been removed with the stomach, duodenum and pancreas an examination is made of the extra-hepatic bile ducts and any tumours or other structures which may be causing adhesions between the liver and the other organs. The duodenum may be slit open so that the orifices of the bile and pancreatic ducts may be examined. Perforating ulcers of the stomach and duodenum are looked for and their exact position and characteristics noted. A probe is gently passed along the bile and the pancreatic ducts as far as possible, to determine their patency and the ducts are then slit up with a probe-pointed bistoury. With a little care, the hepatic duct with its radicles and the cystic duct can be opened up in this manner, and a careful examination made for narrowing, obstruction, inflammation of lining membrane, etc. The portal vein, the hepatic artery and the lymphatic glands in the gastro-hepatic omentum are examined and then the liver is separated from the duodenum and the stomach by cutting through the gastro-hepatic omentum and any adhesions which have formed.

Examination of the liver is now proceeded with.

THE LIVER AND GALL BLADDER.

In a healthy adult the *liver* measures in its transverse diameter from 22 to 30 cm. (9 to 12 ins.) ; in its antero-posterior diameter 17 to 20 cm. (7 to 8 ins.) and in its thickness from above downwards 7 to 9 cm. (3 to $3\frac{1}{2}$ ins.). Its average weight in the male is from 1420 to 1650 grammes (50 to 58 oz.) and in the female 1140 to 1470 grammes (40 to 52 oz.).

The *gall bladder* is about 8 cm. (about 3 ins.) in length and its greatest transverse diameter 2·5 to 3·0 cm. (1 to $1\frac{1}{4}$ ins.).

The weight of the liver should be ascertained.

External examination. Normally the surface of the liver is smooth, but nodular irregularities and grooves are common pathological changes. The grooves are usually shallow and the capsule at the bottom of them is thickened. They are found most commonly in the antero-posterior axis and especially on the upper surface of the right lobe, though not infrequently they may be seen passing transversely across the anterior surface near the lower border. They are really atrophic grooves and generally are produced by pressure on

the liver from without.   The capsule may be thickened generally
and this is characteristic of any atrophic condition affecting
the liver cells, and is, therefore, well marked in cases of acute
and subacute atrophy and of advanced chronic venous congestion.   General thickening of the capsule with adhesions
between it and the diaphragm is sometimes associated with
syphilis.   Localised thickening is often very marked in the
immediate neighbourhood of the gall bladder.

In atrophic conditions the surface of the liver may become
finely granular—a condition frequently seen in advanced cases
of chronic venous congestion—and this is frequently mistaken
for cirrhosis.   Fine granularity of the surface is also seen in
hypertrophic cirrhosis, and coarse granulations are specially
characteristic of atrophic or common cirrhosis, while in syphilis
there may be such irregular scarring that areas of liver tissue
may be more or less completely cut off from the main mass.

Nodules of malignant growths or tumours of other nature,
e.g. angiomas are examined and their general appearances,
their size and their situations noted.

General enlargement of the liver such as is seen in venous
congestion, leucocythæmia, amyloid degeneration, fatty changes,
early alcoholic cirrhosis, hypertrophic, cirrhosis and *local
enlargements* of cancer, suppuration, hydatid cysts, etc. are
always obvious.   The size of the liver, together with accurate
measurements should be recorded, and an outline sketch is
a valuable help in the records of such cases.

Diminution in size, whether local or general, should be noted,
and the weight and measurements ascertained.   The most
common causes of the general reduction in size are advanced
chronic venous congestion, advanced common cirrhosis and
acute or subacute yellow atrophy.

Colour.   Changes in colour are seen in chronic venous
congestion, in which the organ is darker than normal and the
venous channels and central veins of the lobules are prominent
because of their dilatation ; in pernicious anæmia and in hæmochromatosis, in which, owing to a deposit of iron, a brownish
colour is seen; and in fatty changes, especially in fatty infiltration, in which the liver may be canary-yellow in colour.

A greenish colour is seen in catarrhal jaundice, in biliary cirrhosis and in those forms of cancer in which there is interference with the bile passages. In acute yellow atrophy, the reddish and yellow mottling may sometimes be seen on examination of the surface of the liver. Very frequently pale, anæmic-looking patches, of very irregular size, are seen scattered over the liver substance. These are specially marked in livers which are much enlarged and are generally attributed to localised pressure. Minute hæmorrhages may be found under the capsule in cases of toxic poisoning and larger areas of hæmorrhage and actual infarcts are sometimes found.

Consistence. The consistence varies very much, but this is best studied when incisions have been made into its substance. Normally the liver flattens out somewhat after it has been removed from the body, but in cirrhosis of the liver, in chronic venous congestion and particularly in amyloid degeneration the shape is maintained. In the last condition the edges are thickened and rounded and the liver has a firm india-rubber feel.

The *gall bladder* is now opened and the character (colour and viscosity) of the bile is noted, gall stones are looked for, and the mucous membrane is examined. In cases in which there is evidence of cholecystitis and also in typhoid fever or " typhoid carrier " cases, bacteriological examination should be made not only of the contents in the gall bladder but also of the lining membrane.

The liver can be incised in various places and careful examination made of the cut surfaces under the following heads :

Colour and consistence. The friability of the liver is increased in such conditions as poisonings by bacterial products and by some inorganic substances, and in various diseases of the blood, *e.g.* pernicious anæmia. These poisons cause cloudy swelling and fatty changes ; the cells become swollen, the outlines of the lobules are obscured and the surface is paler than normal or has assumed a yellow colour. The degree of these changes varies in different cases. In extreme fatty infiltration the tissue is of a bright canary-yellow colour and the friability is very marked.

The consistence may be increased as a result of distension of the venous channels or as a result of alteration in character or overgrowth of the fibrous tissue stroma.

Thus, in chronic renal congestion, the liver may be very firm though associated fatty changes are usually present ; and this is due to distension of the veins and thickening of their walls. In cirrhosis the increased firmness is due to the overgrowth of fibrous tissue spreading from the portal spaces, and in amyloid degeneration, in which the liver has a gutta-percha-like resistance, the changes are brought about by a great thickening of the fine fibrils in the walls of the blood vessels.

Inspection of the cut surface. Note whether the lobules can be distinctly outlined, whether the central vein is dilated and specially prominent and whether there are any colour changes in the individual lobules. Thus in chronic venous congestion it is often possible to see the dilated and dark central veins of the lobules surrounded by a yellowish ring which is indicative of fatty changes in the cells at the periphery. In more advanced cases irregular reddish and pale areas are seen scattered through the liver substance. The reddish areas represent collections of dilated vessels in situations in which the whole of the liver cells have been destroyed, whereas the pale areas indicate fatty or necrotic changes in the cells which still remain. This mottling of the surface is also seen in cases of acute or subacute yellow atrophy—the red areas again representing dilated vessels, and the pale areas necrotic liver cells.

In amyloid degeneration the tissue is pale and more or less translucent. On the application of a solution of iodine (iodine 1 part, potassium iodide 2 parts, water 100 parts) the amyloid areas become of a deep mahogany brown colour, the unaffected tissues staining yellow. The amyloid material may be patchy in its distribution and then the colour and the consistence of the liver may not be greatly altered from the normal.

In conditions where there is a considerable amount of blood destruction the liver may have a brownish colour owing to the deposition of iron-containing pigments. This is seen in a marked degree in pernicious anæmia, and in hæmochromatosis and to a lesser extent in other diseases where blood destruction is an important feature.   Where the iron is deposited in the form of hæmosiderin, the Prussian blue reaction may be obtained by treating the surface with hydrochloric acid and potassium ferrocyanide (HCl 5% aqueous solution—$K_4FeC_6N_6$ —either a saturated solution, which I prefer or a 10 to 20 % aqueous solution).   The liver tissue may be pigmented in malaria, and the sooty-black pigmentation of melanotic sarcoma may be present in small localised areas or widely spread throughout the liver substance.

Inspection in cases of cirrhosis shews the whitish irregular fibrous tissue and the isolated rather greyish opaque masses of liver cells.   In leucocythæmia and in lymphadenoma, whitish irregular masses may be seen scattered in the liver substance.   The irregular shape and the rather translucent appearance are sufficient to distinguish these from tuberculous nodules—the latter being more rounded and of a dull white colour.   Any abscesses which are present should be described and particular attention given to their situation and their characters.   It is important to observe whether the pus is in the portal vessels, in the bile ducts, or among the liver cells. The character of the contents is noted, whether it is the usual greenish-yellow pus, whether it contains rounded bodies such as one sees in actinomycosis or whether it is the chocolate coloured necrotic tissue of tropical abscess.

Such pus should always be examined microscopically for bacteria, for hooklets or other structures found in hydatid cysts, and for amœbæ.   Cultures should also be made in order to determine, if possible, the causal organism.

The general characters of malignant growths are now more definitely made out and attention should be directed specially to the consistence of these, to the presence of hæmorrhage, to yellowish areas of necrosis and to pigmentation.   The cancerous nodules are firmer than the sarcomatous and hæmorrhage is less common in them.   Pigmentation may be due to the presence of altered blood, to melanin or to bile pigments.

The small rounded areas of necrosis (focal necrosis) which

occur in typhoid fever, diphtheria and other infective diseases should be looked for.

Hydatid cysts, hæmorrhages and infarcts are now examined in more detail and their extent defined. Gummata may be seen and their relation to the scarring which had been noticed on the surface observed.

THE GALL BLADDER.

The general characters of the contents of the gall bladder have already been noted, and any gall stones removed. Examination should now be made in more detail of the mucous membrane to determine the presence of catarrh. In the *acute* cases the membrane is thickened and congested, whereas in the *chronic* forms of the disease the bladder is dilated and its mucous membrane thinned. Chronic inflammatory conditions however sometimes lead to great thickening and contraction of the gall bladder. In cases of typhoid fever a special bacteriological examination should be made, not only of the contents of the gall bladder, but also of its mucous membrane. Tumours should be carefully described and special attention given to their association with gall stones, and if possible their site of origin determined. Direct spread to the liver or secondary growths in the lymphatic glands and in other situations must be looked for, and any evidence of obstruction to the bile-passages or the vessels in the hilus noted. Examination of the character of the gall stones should be made and their numbers, their size and external characters, their appearance in section and, where necessary, their chemical composition ascertained.

THE SPLEEN.

External examination. Size. The normal spleen measures about 11 to 14 cm. (5 ins.) in length, 7 to 8 cm. (3 ins.) in width and 2 to 3 cm. (1 in.) in thickness. Its weight is from 150 to 200 grammes (5 to 7 oz.). There may be various degrees of enlargement or diminution in size as a result of pathological conditions. These should be noted and the measurements and weight of the organ recorded.

Enlargements are found in leucocythæmia, splenic anæmia, malaria, kala-azar, and to a lesser degree in lymphadenoma, tuberculosis, amyloid degeneration, acute congestion, and chronic venous congestion. Diminution in size is common in old age and in general wasting diseases.

Colour and consistence. The healthy spleen is of a brownish-purple colour and in consistence moderately firm. In the majority of acute infective diseases it becomes paler, of a pink tint and very soft, loses its normal shape and becomes flattened out. In some cases where the congestion is very marked the colour may be a deep red. In typhoid fever the softening does not take place and the colour change is not so marked, though in all cases the redness is more evident than in the healthy organ. The absence of softening in this disease is in part due to the great proliferation of the endothelial cells lining the sinuses.

The spleen is dark in colour and very firm in consistence in chronic venous congestion, owing to the distension of the sinuses with venous blood.

In leucocythæmia and in lymphadenoma, there may be very little alteration in colour, though, as a general rule, the organ is paler than normal. The consistence is increased. In malaria the colour is usually dark and the organ either firm or in the more acute cases very soft.

Capsule. Thickening may occur, particularly in cases of enlargement of the organ, and this may be general or may be confined to one surface. Adhesions to the surrounding structures may result from chronic inflammatory or irritative changes. The capsule is usually opaque (due to thickening) and wrinkled in atrophic conditions. Small areas of thickening are sometimes seen scattered over the surface. These are usually irregular in shape and in size and of a glistening white colour. They must be distinguished from acute or chronic miliary tubercles which are of a dull grey colour and are found in the substance of the organ as well as on the surface. The areas of localised thickening may be so marked as to constitute the so-called " flat fibromas." Irregularities of the surface, with occasionally localised thickenings of the capsule are seen in infarction, and in new formations (lymphadenoma and tumours).

Surface irregularities. These may be due to the fibrous nodules already referred to or to miliary tubercles, but larger irregularities are produced by :

(1) *Infarcts.* The base of the infarct is at the surface of the organ, and may be very dark in colour in the early stage or a dull white or pale yellow in the later stage. The area may be irregular in shape, may form a bar across the organ, or be more or less quadrilateral and may be surrounded by a narrow dark zone of congestion. In the late stages of the condition, the pale area may be depressed below the surface or may merely be represented by an irregular depression in which, externally, there is no evidence of necrotic tissue. In some septic infarcts the necrotic tissue may be soft and even purulent. Infarcts are frequently seen in the enlarged spleen of leucocythæmia.

(2) *New formations.* In lymphadenoma, the surface of the spleen is commonly quite smooth, but in certain cases, where the lymphadenomatous tissue is excessive, distinct irregular whitish nodules are seen causing elevations on the surface. Tumours of the spleen are not common, but primary fibromas, chondromas, and osteomas have been recorded and secondary growths of cancer and of sarcoma occur. These tumours are usually evident on the surface of the organ. Cysts due to the *Tænia echinococcus* may also be met with.

The examination of the cut surface. One incision is usually made through the spleen in its long axis, though other incisions may be required under special circumstances.

The points which call for special notice on the cut surface are as follows :

(1) *Colour and consistence.* These features have already been referred to in dealing with the external appearances and they are merely confirmed on examination of the cut surface. The softened pulp is however more obvious and it may be almost fluid in consistence in the acute infective diseases.

The colour of the spleen may be of a distinctly brownish tint and on the application of the Prussian blue test a deep blue or a greenish-blue colour may be produced. This is dependent upon the presence of iron-containing pigment and is associated with all diseases in which blood destruction is a marked feature. In chronic malaria the colour may be very dark owing to a deposit of melanin.

Post-mortem discolouration, giving a greenish or black colour, is usually seen at that part of the spleen which lies in contact with the splenic flexure of the colon.

(2) *Malpighian bodies.* These appear in the healthy spleen as minute pale grey areas about 1 mm. in diameter. In atrophic conditions, *e.g.* in cases in which there is general atrophy or in which the atrophy of the lymphoid tissue is due to pressure from distended venous sinuses or other causes, the Malpighian bodies are reduced in size and may not be visible to the naked eye. Thus in the atrophy of old age or of wasting diseases, and also in cases of advanced chronic venous congestion, the Malpighian bodies may not be seen. Again, in the condition of diffuse waxy degeneration where the walls of the venous sinuses are specially involved, they may not be visible.

More important, however, is the enlargement and greater prominence of the Malpighian bodies. Thus in some cases of acute congestion they become extremely prominent, and of pale or yellowish-grey appearance, whilst in others there is no obvious enlargement, though in these latter the pulp may shew very marked congestion and softening.

In sago-waxy spleen the enlargement and translucent appearance of the Malpighian bodies is the marked feature of the condition and, after pouring some iodine over the surface, they appear more definitely as mahogany-brown nodules. In diffuse waxy spleen the mahogany brown colour is more widely spread, due to the involvement of the walls of the venous sinuses, and the Malpighian bodies may or may not be evident. In leucocythæmia they can usually be made out ; but there may be no obvious enlargement. In lymphadenoma they are irregularly enlarged and project on the cut surface. Scattered over the surface they are seen as greyish irregular nodules, varying much in size and often shewing at their periphery a yellowish pigmented zone. They have been compared very aptly to the pieces of suet seen in a cold suet pudding. In some cases they appear as thick branching processes and masses of irregular nodules. In differentiating these from the tuberculous nodules of acute miliary tuberculosis, the more opaque appearance, and the greater regularity in shape and size of the latter are of importance, but the fact that numbers of the tubercle granulations can be seen in the subcapsular region on external examination of the spleen is of special diagnostic value, for in lymphadenoma the subcapsular lymphatics are either completely devoid of nodules or if these are present they appear as large irregular masses resembling new growths.

The larger tuberculous masses, " ape tuberculosis," nearly always shew caseation and softening in their centres and are not likely to be mistaken for lymphadenomatous nodules.

(3) *Infarcts*. Their characters are now seen more definitely and note is made of their shape, their colour, and any evidences of softening or calcification. The peripheral zone is examined for congestion or for fibrous tissue, and the vessels are examined for evidences of thrombosis or embolism.

(4) *New growths*. Tumours and cysts are more clearly defined and their general appearances described.

Portions of the organ are now removed for histological examination, the part from which the blocks are taken being determined by the pathological condition found in the organ.

Spleniculi are often found in the neighbourhood of the spleen, and these will generally be found to shew the same changes as those found in the spleen itself.

THE KIDNEYS AND SUPRARENALS.

Shennan gives the following as the average weight of the kidneys :

Males.	Left kidney	182	grammes	($6\frac{1}{2}$ oz.)
	Right kidney	181	,,	($6\frac{2}{5}$ oz.)
Females.	Left kidney	152·5	,,	($5\frac{2}{5}$ oz.)
	Right kidney	151	,,	($5\frac{1}{3}$ oz.).

For all practical purposes the weight of each kidney in the male may be taken as 182 grammes (6½ oz.) and in the female 151 grammes (5⅓ oz.). The average length is 11–12 cm. (4½ ins.), the width about 5–6 cm. (2 ins.) and thickness 3–4 cm. (1¼ ins.).

The examination should be carried out in the following order :

(1) *Shape and size. Enlargement* of the kidney is shewn not only by an increase in length but very commonly by an increase in thickness. Such enlargements are seen in most acute and subacute inflammatory conditions, in amyloid degeneration and in many cases where there are extensive fatty changes, and, in such conditions, the enlargement is usually uniform and both kidneys are affected almost equally.

The majority of new growths produce enlargements, which are more or less localised and frequently confined to one kidney. Considerable enlargement of one kidney is sometimes seen in association with atrophy, with congenital defect or with absence of the opposite kidney.   In the condition of *congenital cystic kidney* both organs are enlarged.

Diminution in size is seen in congenital conditions, in atrophy from disease, *e.g.* granular contracted kidney, or from loss of function, *e.g.* by impaction of a calculus, and there is always some reduction in size in the late stages of chronic nephritis.

Measurements and weights should be recorded.

Alterations in shape are not of special importance.   They are seen particularly in cases of new growth, but may also be associated with chronic inflammatory changes in the kidney.

Congenital alterations such as " horse-shoe " kidney should be observed, and in such cases careful notes made of any abnormalities in the blood supply or in the ureters.   The bridge joining the kidneys is usually at the lower end and the ureters pass down in front of the bridge.   The ureters may be double throughout, or the two tubes may coalesce at any level in the lower part of their course.

In all cases of congenital abnormalities, special examination should be made of the genital apparatus.   This is of the greatest importance in cases where one kidney is absent or where it is very small.   The ureter may be absent or present in such cases and may be patent or closed at one end.   It is not uncommon to get abnormal branches arising from the renal artery.   Note should be made of all such abnormalities.

(2)   *Colour and consistence.* The healthy kidney is of a reddish-brown colour, and firm in consistence.   In acute diseases, *e.g.* cloudy swelling, acute nephritis, and fatty degeneration, where there is swelling of the parenchymatous tissue associated with necrotic changes in the cells, the organ is *paler* than normal and in cases where fatty degeneration becomes marked it assumes a *yellow* colour.   In amyloid degeneration, the pallor is very marked and the consistence increased.   Pallor is also a well marked feature in some cases of subacute and chronic nephritis, *e.g.* the, badly named, " large white kidney " and the " small white kidney."   Thus it will be seen that pallor of the kidney substance is associated with various very dissimilar pathological conditions, and little dependence can be placed upon it in diagnosis.

In chronic venous congestion the kidney becomes of a bluish-purple colour, and the consistence is greatly increased owing to the distension of the whole venous system of the organ. In cases of thrombosis of the renal artery or of a main branch, the whole kidney or the part supplied by the branch, becomes engorged with blood and assumes a dark reddish colour.   In some forms of chronic nephritis associated with arterio-sclerotic changes, the kidney substance becomes redder than normal— " small red kidney."   The consistence is always increased in chronic inflammatory or chronic degenerative conditions, owing partly to atrophy of the secreting structures and partly to an overgrowth of fibrous tissue.

Local colour changes which result from petechial or larger hæmorrhages, from tumour growths, from infarctions and from infiltrations and degenerations of various kinds will be best dealt with after the capsule has been stripped and described.

The greenish colour due to bile pigments, the yellowish-brown colour seen in cases of extensive blood destruction, *e.g.* hæmoglobinuria and hæmochromatosis, and the bluish-green appearance of decomposition, are so obvious that it is hardly necessary to draw attention to them.

(3) *The capsule.* In the healthy kidney the capsule is translucent ; and, though, in certain cases, it may be slightly adherent along the grooves which still mark the fœtal lobulation, it, as a general rule, strips easily leaving a smooth surface. In pathological conditions the capsule may be thickened and opaque, and firmly adherent not only to the kidney substance, but also to the perinephric tissues. These changes are specially seen in those cases of chronic nephritis or chronic arterial degeneration, in which the kidney is atrophied. The perinephric fat is increased in amount, and usually firmly adherent to the capsule of the kidney. To examine the capsule completely a section must be made of the kidney. To do this the kidney is held firmly in the left hand between the fingers and thumb—the convex border projecting outwards. With the left kidney the anterior (ventral) surface, and, with the right kidney, the posterior (dorsal) surface will lie against the thumb and thenar eminence. With a sharp, long-bladed knife, an incision is made in the longitudinal axis of the kidney extending from pole to pole and from the convex border to the hilus. Gripping the capsule at the cut surface either between the forefinger and thumb of the right hand or with a pair of dissecting forceps, it is stripped backwards to the hilus on each half of the organ. Note is now made as to whether it strips easily, whether it is slightly adherent at certain areas or whether it is adherent over the whole surface, and whether, in the process of separation, part of the kidney substance comes away with the capsule. It should be noted that in some cases where the capsule is thickened, a superficial layer may be stripped, the deeper part still remaining attached to the kidney. Care therefore should be taken that the whole of the layers of the capsule have been stripped in estimating the degree of adhesion.

(4) *The surface of the kidney.* Normally this should be smooth, though, in many cases, irregular sulci are seen scattered over the surface—the remains of the fœtal lobulation. In some

pathological conditions, even of a gross character, this smoothness of the surface may be retained, whilst in others the surface may be irregularly granular or may shew a greater or less degree of scarring. The granularity is characteristic of marked arterial degeneration and also is secondary to inflammatory changes (granular contracted kidney). A coarse granulation is sometimes seen in cases of amyloid degeneration with marked interstitial changes. Irregular scars are a common result of advanced interstitial changes, especially those cases in which the fibrous tissue is patchy in its distribution, and in cases where there have been infarcts which have become partially absorbed, scars are produced.

Cysts. An irregularity of the surface due to the large cysts of congenital cystic kidneys is obvious. Numerous cysts, varying much in size and in colour, are common in cases of chronic nephritis. These may be very small and, in stripping the capsule, they may be torn and may appear on the surface as minute depressions. Larger cystic dilatations due to blocking of the ureter, to tuberculosis of the kidney, or to septic pyelonephrosis, may give the surface a very irregular appearance.

Hæmorrhages. Minute hæmorrhages are common in cases of toxic poisoning and also in cases of acute and subacute nephritis. Larger hæmorrhages are less common, but I have seen very extensive hæmorrhage under the capsule of the kidney and in its substance as a result of the rupture of minute aneurisms.

Infarcts. These usually appear on the surface of the kidney as irregular pale areas raised above or depressed below the general surface, and surrounded by a zone of congestion. In the later stages, they may be represented by irregular scars.

Tumours and other new formations in the kidney may of course appear on the surface as regular or irregular masses, usually of a pale colour. Miliary tubercles and small abscesses may be seen, syphilitic gummata sometimes occur, and nodules of lymphatic tissue, sometimes forming masses $\frac{1}{8}$ to $\frac{1}{4}$ in. in diameter, are observed in some cases of lymphatic leukæmia.

These latter usually shew more or less hæmorrhage into their substance.

Colour. The changes in colour which were noticed before the capsule was stripped are again observed.

(5) *Examination of the cut surface of the kidney.* Evidence of the cysts, hæmorrhages, infarcts, tumours and other new growths, which have been noted in the examination of the surface, is again seen, and a more detailed description as to site, extent and general characters of these pathological conditions can be given.

Special attention, however, should be directed to the following points :

(a) *The cortex.* Relative thickness of the superficial part of the cortex to the medulla. In the normal kidney the superficial cortex is about one-third of the width of the medulla, but as the medulla undergoes comparatively little change in diseased conditions, changes in the cortex are usually very obvious. These are of the nature of swelling and thickening or atrophy and narrowing so that the normal proportions between the two parts are altered. The interpyramidal cortex shews the same changes as are seen in the superficial cortex, though usually not to the same degree. Again, on close examination of the normal cortex, it is seen to be made up of pale columns separated by darker lines all running parallel to one another and perpendicularly to the surface. The pale, somewhat translucent, columns represent the tubules and the dark lines the blood vessels (Pl. VI fig. 10). In those diseased conditions where the main affection is a swelling of the cells of the secreting tubules the pale columns become thickened and opaque and may assume a dull grey or yellow colour, whereas in cases in which the vessels are specially dilated (*e.g.* chronic venous congestion), the dark lines stand out prominently. The regularity of these columns and lines is of special importance, for, where there is an overgrowth of fibrous tissue in the cortex, a marked distortion of both the vessels and the tubules takes place, and these " markings " in the cortex become very irregular. Normally the Malpighian bodies are not seen with the naked eye, but in conditions where there is much distension of the

Plate VI

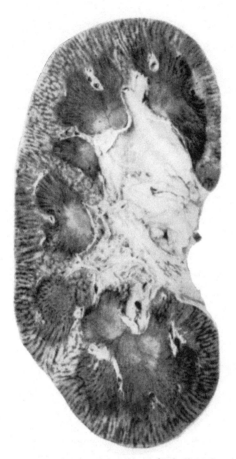

Fig. 10. Kidney, shewing the vascular markings (dark lines in cortex) and tubules (pale areas between the dark lines). Note also the straight vessels in the pyramids. The dark lines in the cortex become distorted when interstitial changes are present and the pale areas are thickened where swelling of the cells of the tubules is present.

glomerular tuft (*e.g.* in chronic venous congestion) or where the fibrous tissue of the walls is much thickened (*e.g.* in amyloid degeneration) they may become prominent as dark or as more or less translucent points.

From what has been said above, it will be clear that the conditions in which swelling of the cortex is a prominent feature are those in which poisons act acutely or subacutely on the secreting cells, causing them to undergo cloudy swelling and the consequent changes of fatty degeneration and necrosis; or those in which there is considerable distension in the inter-lobular vessels and glomerular capillaries, or thickening of the fibrous tissue in the walls of these vessels. Thickening of the cortex occurs, therefore, in acute and in subacute parenchymatous nephritis, in cloudy swelling and in fatty degeneration resulting from general toxic poisoning, in the large form of amyloid kidney and in cases of chronic venous congestion.

Diminution in the size of the cortex occurs particularly in atrophic conditions which are associated with an impaired blood supply and in cases where there have been long-standing chronic inflammatory or irritative changes producing an overgrowth of fibrous tissue. Thus, in the various forms of granular contracted kidney, the atrophy of the cortex is a marked feature and in cases of chronic interstitial nephritis similar changes are seen.

(*b*) *The medulla.* The changes in the pyramids are not of special importance, though in chronic venous congestion the straight vessels may be dilated and very prominent, and, in other conditions, casts or deposits of salts (such as urates) may be seen in the collecting tubules. Infarcts in the medulla are uncommon. Pus is sometimes seen in the tubules.

(*c*) *The renal pelvis.* Search should be made for any evidence of catarrhal or inflammatory changes in the mucous membrane, for hæmorrhage and for calculi. If dilatation is present (hydronephrosis), its degree should be noted and search made for its cause, and therefore the ureter, the bladder and the urethra should be carefully examined for calculi, inflammatory or other causes of stricture, tuberculosis, suppuration, etc.

Suppuration. There may be definite abscesses in any part

of the kidney substance or, as is stated above, accumulations of pus may be found in the renal pelvis and in the dilated calyces. In some cases the kidney substance may be so extensively atrophied that the organ is converted into a bag of pus. More important, however, is the observation of the extension of purulent affections into the kidney substance along the lines of the tubules or the vessels, without evidence of dilatation of the renal pelvis and without the formation of large abscesses. In these cases, the pus shews itself as pale yellowish lines in the pyramids or in the cortex, these lines being in the course of the vessels or the tubules. In such cases a greater or a smaller number of minute yellowish points surrounded by a red congested zone are seen on the surface of the kidney.

Tuberculosis. This may be evidenced by the presence of small grey miliary tubercles, both on the surface and on the cut section, or by a more extensive tuberculous infiltration which may involve the pelvis and calyces, so that the kidney substance may be almost completely destroyed. In such cases the walls of the dilated calyces and pelvis are lined with caseous material. Examination should also be made of the ureter, bladder, vas deferens, vesiculæ seminales and testes.

Cysts. Reference has already been made to cysts on the surface and on section, and usually it is sufficient in notes of the examination to indicate their presence, but sometimes the character of the contents may require to be noted. This is particularly the case in larger cysts, *e.g.* those due to echinococcus.

Tumours. The site, the size and the general characteristics of tumours will of course be noted. The majority of these will not escape the observation of the pathologist, but very small tumours in the pyramids, such as fibromata, may easily be missed.

Pigmentation. General alterations in colour due to the presence of fat, of iron-containing pigments, and those associated with such conditions as chronic venous congestion, atrophic and inflammatory conditions have already been referred to. Localised pigmented areas may occur as in melanotic sarcomas and in " argyria."

(*d*) *Vessels*. The larger renal vessels should be examined for thrombosis and atheroma and the small vessels which are seen on the cut surface of the kidney often give indication of arterial degeneration by their thickened walls and open mouths.

Nephritis (inflammatory and degenerative conditions in the kidney). Much information may be obtained as to the presence of nephritis in either its acute or chronic form by observing the size, colour, and appearance of the surface and of the section of the kidney, in the manner already described, but the pathologist who depends upon these for a diagnosis must in a considerable proportion of cases give an erroneous report. Microscopical examination is essential and therefore I feel that it would not only be useless, but also misleading to refer further to naked eye appearance of the kidney in a book which has for its aim such instruction as will be helpful to the pathologist in his methods of operating and which will also give him some general idea of the appearances of the organs in the pathological conditions for which he must be on the outlook. As has been said, microscopical examination is essential, and in cases of nephritis, especially, no definite opinion should be given until the microscopical sections have been carefully examined.

Certain clinical manifestations such as hæmorrhage, and certain obvious pathological conditions which have as their causal factor something outside the kidney itself, *e.g.* hydronephrosis, some forms of tuberculosis, etc., will be dealt with separately in a later chapter.

The Suprarenals.

It is not common to find diseased conditions in the suprarenals, but their examination should never be omitted. They may be entirely absent, or only fragments of tissue corresponding to them may be present. The gross pathological lesions are so few and so obvious that a pathologist can generally have no doubt as to the condition he is dealing with. In Addison's disease, of course, special attention must be directed to the examination of the suprarenals for tuberculosis, for fibrosis, or for atrophy. Syphilitic gummata may occur and amyloid degeneration is not infrequent. Hæmorrhage into the suprarenal should always indicate a special search for the cause. It is found in leucocythæmia and possibly in other blood diseases, whilst in some toxic poisonings small hæmorrhages may be found. Traumatism, such as fracture of the spine, rupture of the liver, etc., may cause injury to the suprarenal. Cases of hæmorrhage may occur, and recently I have seen at least two, where no obvious cause could be found, and where no other gross pathological lesion was present.

Tumours of the suprarenal should be very carefully examined and described, but no decision should be given as to their nature without microscopical examination. It is always important to remember that the tumours may be bilateral—both organs suffering almost to an equal extent.

Accessory suprarenals, or at any rate structures resembling in many respects suprarenal tissue, and in some cases developmentally related to the suprarenals, are sometimes found in the mesentery, in the broad ligament, on the ovarian or spermatic vessels, in the vaginal walls, in the inguinal canal, in the epididymis, or embedded in the kidney, the liver or the pancreas.

Sexual abnormalities such as a growth of hair on the pubis in young children or an excessive growth of hair on the face in women should always direct attention to the suprarenals. Ernest Glynn and others have shewn that tumours of the cortical portions in the suprarenals are sometimes associated with sex abnormalities, and, in association with changes in the suprarenal, pathological conditions may occur in the pituitary body.

STOMACH, DUODENUM AND PANCREAS.

On *external* examination attention is directed specially to the shape of the stomach, its size, the condition of the glands in the lesser curvature, the presence of any ulcers which have perforated and the presence of any tumour visible or palpable from the outside. The duodenum is specially examined for ulcers and the pancreas for tumours, for cirrhotic conditions, for acute inflammatory and hæmorrhagic conditions and for any evidence of necrosis.

The shape of the stomach. Hour glass contraction of the stomach is the most common deformity, and when this is observed, the following points need special attention.

(1) Is this condition merely the result of rigor mortis or is it a definite pathological one ?

If the cause be merely rigor mortis, the apparent contraction can be completely removed by distending the stomach with water, whereas, if it is pathological the contracted portion will not be altered to any marked degree by this mechanical process.

(2) Sometimes, though rarely, the first part of the duodenum becomes distended as a result of stricture in the region of Vater's ampulla and in one case which I saw there was a definite malignant growth apparently taking its origin at the bile papilla. Such cases are apt to be mistaken for hour glass contraction of the stomach.

The size of the stomach. This is best estimated by measuring the capacity of the organ when moderately distended. In the adult it will hold 1000 c.c. (35 to 40 oz.). The abnormally distended stomach is usually so altered in shape that measurements in length or in width are not of much value. Before measurements of capacity are made the contents of the stomach should be poured out through the cut œsophagus into a clean glass vessel, and note made of their general characteristics. By following this plan the presence of blood, of necrotic tissue and of foreign bodies, etc. is detected. In medico-legal cases the contents should be preserved for future examination.

Opening the stomach and duodenum. With a pair of blunt-pointed scissors, a curved incision is made starting at the anterior surface of the œsophagus and passing along the anterior surface of the stomach, about 1 in. above the greater curvature, through the pylorus and duodenum. Before cutting through the pylorus, the cardiac side of it should as far as possible be examined through the opening already made, for ulceration, etc., and the finger passed through the pyloric ring to detect any evidence of stenosis. With the forefinger through the ring and the thumb outside, any evidence of thickness or induration should be examined for.

Points to be looked for in the opened œsophagus, stomach and duodenum.

(1) *Post-mortem digestion.* This condition is common, especially in young children, and must be carefully distinguished from ulceration. Post-mortem digestion is found especially in that part of the stomach on which the food lies when the body is lying in the prone position. The mucous membrane alone may be involved and becomes swollen, soft and translucent, or the condition may spread more deeply into the muscular coat. The position, the extent of the destructive changes, the irregularity of the edges and the absence of any sign of inflammation are usually sufficient to differentiate it from ulceration.

(2) *Colour changes in the mucous membrane.* In cases where there has been venous congestion or chronic catarrh, the decomposition changes may make the mucous membrane dark green or black, from the action of sulphuretted hydrogen on the iron-containing pigments which have been deposited in the tissues. In acute catarrhal conditions, the mucous membrane may assume a pinkish colour and in addition there may be numerous petechial hæmorrhages scattered over the surface. These areas of hæmorrhage should be specially examined for evidence of ulceration.

(3) *Evidence of ulceration* should be carefully looked for. The ordinary, well-defined, peptic ulcer is not likely to be missed, but the scars of former ulcers and particularly minute ulcers and so-called hæmorrhagic erosions are very frequently overlooked and the greatest care should be exercised in examining for them. The latter may be hidden by the rugæ, or owing to contraction of the stomach, they may be almost completely obliterated. Only a systematic and careful examination of the whole mucous membrane can justify the conclusion that such minute ulcers are absent. In cases where there has

been hæmatemesis it is specially important that this careful examination of the mucous membrane be made. Where large ulcers are found, the blood vessels must be examined for evidence of thrombosis, and the edges and floor carefully palpated for any induration which may suggest malignant disease. In all cases it is very important that a careful histological examination be made of several portions of tissue removed from the ulcerated area, before concluding that malignant disease is absent. Ulceration due to *B. tuberculosis* or *B. typhosus* is extremely rare in the stomach. In cases of general chronic venous congestion and particularly in portal obstruction, the walls of the stomach, particularly the mucous and submucous coats, are thickened, the inner surface is of a brownish or slaty-blue colour ; small ulcers are common, especially on the summits of the ridges of the mucous membrane and, particularly in cases of portal obstruction, there is a varicose condition of the venous plexus at the lower end of the œsophagus. It is important to note these varicose veins and the small ulcers because from them hæmorrhages frequently occur, and I think it is not too much to say, that in the vast majority of cases of hæmorrhage from the stomach, if not in all, some definite pathological lesion here or elsewhere in the organ will be found if it is looked for with sufficient care.

(4) *Tumours of the stomach.* Tumours of the stomach are usually so obvious that it is hardly necessary to do more than mention them. Their exact structure can only be determined by histological examination, which should always be undertaken ; but in some cases naked eye appearances may be sufficient to give some indication as to the nature of the growth. The hard, fibrous structure of the scirrhus cancer, the soft spongy feel of the medullary form, and the gelatinous appearance of the colloid type, are usually important indications of the nature of the growth, but these appearances do not justify a neglect of histological examination. Carcinoma is the common tumour of the stomach, sarcoma is rare. Simple tumours, such as fibromata, myomata and fibro-myomata, occur. Gummata may occur and lymphomatous nodules have been described. Microscopical examination alone can

determine the nature of such growths.　In tumours about the pylorus there may be a considerable amount of fibrous tissue and, recently, several observers have attributed many of the strictures of the pylorus to fibrosis rather than to cancer. In such cases therefore it is essential that histological examination should be made, not at one part only, but at several areas, for one area may give evidence of fibrosis only, whereas another may shew the cells of cancer.

(5)　*Inflammatory conditions of the stomach.*　The pathologist must always recognise that the naked eye appearances of acute inflammation of the stomach are very soon altered after death, partly by digestion and partly by decomposition, and that in a considerable proportion of cases very little information of value is obtained.　If the organ is examined very soon after death, the mucous membrane is swollen, diffusely congested, and frequently shews minute hæmorrhages, and the glands are specially active so that the surface becomes covered with a glairy tenacious mucous.　These appearances are of special importance in dealing with cases of food poisoning.　In the more chronic cases there is a slaty-grey discolouration and the mucous membrane may be atrophied.　Follicular ulcers are common.　Great thickening of the walls of the stomach due to diffuse inflammatory and suppurative changes in the sub-mucous coat is found in cases of phlegmonous gastritis, and in such conditions a bacteriological examination is essential. Membranous gastritis is very rare.

DUODENUM AND PANCREAS.

Duodenum.　The duodenal papilla should be sought and a probe passed into the pancreatic duct to decide as to its patency. Dilatation of the duodenum should be noted and any evidence of old or recent ulcers looked for.　Tumours are not common but may be found starting from the papilla.　Any signs of inflammation must be noted.

The pancreas.　Softening of the pancreas is common, probably as a result of digestion with its secretion, and, especially in microscopical examination, it is important to guard against confusing this condition with necrosis. The duct has already been examined from the duodenal opening for patency, and this examination should now be continued by slitting open the duct into which a grooved director has been placed. Calculi are to be looked for. Injuries or disease of the pancreas, which enable its secretion to escape either into its substance or into the peritoneal cavity, are at once recognised by masses of irregular dull whitish areas in the glandular tissue or in the fat in the neighbourhood—" fat necrosis."

Acute inflammatory conditions, such as acute hæmorrhagic pancreatitis, give rise to great softening of the organ with more or less hæmorrhage and evidence of fat necrosis. There is usually no difficulty in recognising such condition at the post-mortem examination.

Interstitial overgrowth—fibrosis—in the pancreas must always be looked for, and it is important to remember that the fibrosis may be quite local. In diabetes mellitus, a special examination is made of the pancreas for any pathological condition, but especially for fibrosis. Histological examination is essential in all cases, attention being directed to evidence of necrosis, hyaline degeneration, and fibrosis. The condition of the islets of Langerhans is of great importance and particularly any evidence of atrophy or fibrosis of these. Tumours of the pancreas usually present no difficulties, but in all cases where the site is at or near the head, careful examination should be made of the glands there. Carcinoma is the most common form of growth.

Other pathological conditions of the pancreas which should be borne in mind in conducting an autopsy are, tuberculosis which is rare, syphilis, which causes fibrosis and periarteritis and sometimes gummata, and cysts. The latter may be moderately large or they may be small and multiple. The multiple cysts are rare and are usually associated with cysts in the liver and in the kidney.

Accessory pancreases are sometimes found in the wall of the stomach, duodenum, jejunum and in other situations. They are not of special pathological importance.

The Intestine.

A general examination of the external surface of the intestine should be made with the special object of detecting any evidence of stricture, of localised dilatation, localised peritonitis or old adhesions, and of diverticula, and note should be made of the exact site, extent and nature of these. The strictures may be due to malignant disease, to tuberculous disease, to bands of adhesions or to fibrosis, and evidence of their exact nature may be sometimes obtained on external examination alone. The dilatations are usually observed before the intestines have been removed, but their exact site is often more definitely made out after removal. They are most commonly found above strictures, though in carcinoma of the rectum the dilatation is frequently found below and not above the seat of the stricture. The most marked dilatation which occurs is that of the colon in Hirschsprung's disease. It must always be remembered that paralytic distension of the intestine is common and that no evidence of any pathological causal condition may be found. Strictures also result during the " death period " from rigor mortis and in such cases the bowel is easily distended with fluid.

Of diverticula, the most common is Meckel's. It varies much in length and occurs about 60 cm. (2 feet) above the ileo-cœcal valve. Smaller diverticula, particularly in the mesenteric attachment of the small intestine, are more likely to be missed. These, not uncommonly, have portions of aberrant pancreatic tissue at their apices. In the large intestine diverticula are also found but these are usually merely due to distension of the normal sacculations and frequently contain scybalous masses.

Examination of the interior of the intestine. Divide the small from the large intestine by cutting through the former about 2 ins. above the ileo-cœcal valve, and then the usual practice is to wash out the intestinal contents with a stream of running water and to slit open the bowel and examine the mucous membrane. This certainly is the cleanest method of procedure but it has the disadvantage of disturbing the relations of the contents and where permanent specimens are required it is extremely difficult to fix the colour after much washing. In most cases the disturbing of the relations of the contents is not of much importance and in these cases if the intestine is put into Jores', Pick's, Kaiserling's, or other preserving fluid for some minutes before it is washed, the subsequent washing does little harm and the colours can be quite readily retained in permanent specimens. In cases where the relations of the contents are of importance, the bowel must be opened without being washed out and the operator will find it very desirable to wear rubber gloves, as it is difficult to rid the hands of the penetrating odour of the fæces.

When the contents are washed out before the bowel is opened, the washings should be collected into some vessels and carefully examined for parasites or other abnormalities. Having washed out the intestine or having decided that the washing out is not desirable, the blunt point of the bowel scissors is introduced into the small intestine, and, with the left hand the intestine is rapidly drawn over the blade of the scissors, which are held in the right hand with the blades at an acute angle. When getting a new grip on the intestine with the left hand the bowel is apt to slip off the blade of the scissors and, it is in order to prevent this, that I prefer the scissors with the slightly recurved point, which catch the bowel as it is slipping backwards. The incision should be made along the line of the mesenteric attachment and if the intestine has been carefully removed from the body, so that there are no kinks in it, due to mesenteric attachments, the operation is an extremely simple one, and especially if the bowel is allowed to remain partially distended with water.

The large intestine is opened in a similar manner, the line of incision being along one of the longitudinal bands of muscle. One generally finds that the scissors have to be used more in the ordinary cutting fashion in the large intestine, especially when opening the cæcum, than in the small intestine.

The whole of the mucous membrane is now carefully examined, and this is most conveniently done by pulling the intestine between the ring and middle finger and over the forefinger of the left hand.

The points to which attention should be given are :

(1) *Inflammatory changes.* The appearances of these are usually so altered by post-mortem digestion, etc. that little importance can be attached to mere naked eye examination. Hæmorrhages may be evident and the mucous membrane may be thickened and covered with tenacious mucous. The lymphoid nodules may be considerably swollen, especially in the large intestine and in some cases a definite membrane may have formed. In the more chronic forms the mucous membrane may shew a brownish or greyish discolouration.

(2) *Ulceration.* Follicular ulceration is very common in catarrhal conditions and is usually associated with swollen follicles. The larger irregular ulcers of typhoid fever and of tuberculosis, and the extensive ulceration of colitis and of dysentery can hardly be overlooked. In describing the ulcers, their situation, their size, their general characters, especially as to the character of their margins and their floors, and their relation to the Peyer's patches and solitary glands, should be carefully noted. The associated changes in the wall of the intestine, such as the thickening in cases of dysentery, the infiltration in tuberculosis, and the contraction and stricture in tuberculosis, in syphilis and in malignant disease, should be looked for.

(3) *Tumours of the intestine.* These again usually present no difficulty to the pathologist. He simply has to note their situation and their general characters, but for their nature he will necessarily depend on a microscopical examination, though his general knowledge will frequently enable him to say at once whether the tumour is a malignant or a simple one, and even to give an opinion as to the type of the tumour. The simple tumours, myoma, fibroma, lipoma and adenoma are quite unimportant. Of the malignant tumours the columnar-celled, spheroidal-celled and colloid cancers are the most common. Squamous epitheliomata may develop at the lower end of the rectum. Sarcomata are very rare.

CHAPTER VI

EXAMINATION OF CERVICAL AND MEDIASTINAL TISSUES

Cervical and mediastinal tissues. (Mouth, pharynx, larynx, trachea, œsophagus, thyroid, thymus, cervical glands. etc.)

Unless the post-mortem is a restricted one, these tissues will be removed either in connection with the thoracic organs or after the lungs and the heart have been removed. The latter will be the method usually followed.

A general examination of the tissues should at first be made and any pathological changes, such as enlargement or atrophy of glands, presence of new growths, recorded.

The tissues should then be placed on a table with the œsophagus uppermost and the opening of the larynx pointing to the operator. With blunt-pointed scissors the œsophagus and the pharynx should be slit open from the lower to the upper end. The condition of the mucous membrane, such as erosion or staining from irritant poisons or other causes, the presence of stricture or dilatation, of new growths and of dilated and varicose veins at the lower end, should be examined.

The conditions due to poisons will be dealt with in Chapter XI. Stricture may be due to compression from without by tumours or aneurisms and may not be evident at this stage of the examination ; or it may be caused by the impaction of foreign bodies, by the presence of tumours or by cicatricial contraction due to damage to the wall by corrosives, by boiling liquids, etc.

Naked eye examination may be sufficient to indicate the cause, but in many cases microscopical examination will be necessary to enable a positive opinion to be given and in all cases where tumours or fibrous thickenings are present microscopical examination must be made. Ulcers are rare in the œsophagus but may give rise to stricture. Post-mortem digestion which may occur on the posterior wall of the œsophagus must not be mistaken for ulceration. As this condition is more common in the stomach it will be referred to in dealing with the examination of the abdominal organs. Dilatation is not of great importance and is usually secondary to stricture.

Of the new growths the most common is squamous-celled carcinoma, but other types of cancer may occur, and a microscopical examination should always be made. Simple tumours are not common.

Rarely one finds in the œsophagus a continuation from the mouth of "thrush" (oïdium albicans). Varicose and dilated veins are found at the lower end of the œsophagus in cases of portal obstruction, especially in cirrhosis of the liver, and may give rise to hæmorrhage. They are usually just at the cardiac end of the œsophagus and are perhaps best examined with the stomach.

Tongue, pharynx, larynx and trachea. With a pair of blunt-pointed scissors a mesial incision is made through the posterior wall of the larynx and trachea into the remaining parts of the large bronchi. Grasping the cut surfaces of the larynx in either hand it is gently forced open. No important damage is done by this procedure and the larynx can be more thoroughly inspected.

Examination is now made of the tongue, the tonsils, the retro-pharyngeal tissues, the epiglottis, the vocal cords, the larynx, the trachea and the bronchi.

The tongue. The main pathological changes which require attention in the tongue are the presence of patches of thrush, erosions or ulcers and particularly new growths. Syphilitic gummata may occur and these must be carefully differentiated from tumours, of which the most common is squamous epithelioma. Small blood tumours may be found and abscesses due to the *S. actinomyces* sometimes occur. Diagnosis in such cases can only be satisfactorily made on microscopical examination.

The tonsils and other pharyngeal tissues Special attention is directed to the size of the tonsils and the amount of adenoid tissue (adenoids) present in other parts of the pharynx. The presence of congestion, small or large ulcers, the deposit of membrane and the character of this should be noted. The tonsils should be incised in order to detect any suppurative foci, which are sometimes the primary affection in cases of pyæmia. If retro-pharyngeal suppuration is present it will have already been detected and search should be made for some causal factor. The condition may arise as an affection of the retro-pharyngeal glands secondary to a " septic throat " whether this be associated with diphtheria, scarlet-fever or other cause ; it may be due to a secondary infection from tuberculous or other disease of the cervical vertebræ ; to infection of the mucous membrane and its subjacent tissues as a result of burns, scalds or of the action of corrosives ; to mechanical injury by fish bones, etc. or to suppuration in the middle ear.

Sometimes ulceration resulting from syphilis is seen but this is comparatively rare in the post-mortem room. Tumours are not common but if present they should be examined histologically. Obvious tuberculosis of the tonsils is rare, but microscopical examination often reveals the presence of distinct tuberculous foci, and therefore in any case with enlarged cervical glands or glands about the angle of the jaw, careful microscopical examination should be made of the tonsils.

The epiglottis. This often shares in the diseases of the larynx, and therefore may shew œdema, tuberculous or syphilitic ulceration, etc.

The larynx. This should be examined for stenosis due to pressure from without or to cicatricial contraction from ulcers within. Congestion of the mucous membrane may be seen but is not an important pathological change. Œdema may be present, but this may largely disappear after death and especially after removal of the tissues from the body. Acute laryngitis is not very evident after death, for the congestion and redness may have disappeared. Minute erosions on the vocal cords indicate an acute inflammatory process, while thickening of the mucous membrane with hypertrophy of lymphoid tissue and distension of mucous glands giving the surface a granular appearance is characteristic of chronic inflammation. Membranous deposits due to diphtheria, to other septic infections or to the action of corrosives, etc. should always be examined bacteriologically. Where pus is seen very careful examination should be made for any evidence of perichondritis and of necrosis of the cartilages. Note should be made of the cartilages which are specially affected. The arytenoids are the most commonly involved in the first instance, and the cricoid and thyroid may be attacked secondarily. The pus in such cases should be examined bacteriologically. The condition is most usual in cases of tuberculosis or in syphilis, but may occur in typhoid fever and much more rarely in other conditions.

In cases of tuberculosis and of syphilis of the larynx, examination of special regions is of great importance, *e.g.* in tuberculosis, the arytenoid cartilages and the mucous membrane at their bases, and in syphilis, the base of the epiglottis, but these points will be dealt with in more detail later.

Lupus sometimes affects the larynx and the nodules and the ulcers are most obvious at the margins of the epiglottis or on both its surfaces, though the condition may extend over the aryteno-epiglottic folds on to the surface of the larynx.

Nodules due to leprosy, to glanders or to lymphatic leukæmia may be found in the larynx. The clinical history of the case gives the clue to the condition, and microscopical or bacteriological examination may be necessary to make a positive diagnosis possible.

Tumours of the larynx must be accurately described. The most common are papillomata and squamous epitheliomata.

Trachea. The main points for examination in the trachea are whether there has been an extension to this tube of the conditions seen in the larynx, *e.g.* acute and chronic inflammatory changes, diphtheria, syphilitic and tuberculous ulceration, or whether these conditions exist independently in the trachea. Tuberculous ulceration is generally found on the posterior wall at the upper or lower end of the tube, while syphilitic ulceration is chiefly near the bifurcation and is very generally associated with syphilis in the larynx.

Destruction of the wall of the larynx may be caused by ulceration or infiltration by malignant tumours, by pressure of an aneurism, by softening due to a suppurating gland in contact with the trachea or by syphilitic ulceration.

The anterior surface of these cervical tissues is now examined with special reference to the thyroid and thymus.

Thyroid. If the organ is *enlarged*, its measurements should be taken and special observation made as to whether the enlargement is general or is localised to one special lobe or part of a lobe. The general consistence should be noted and then an incision made into the gland at various points and the cut surface examined.

The principal conditions which give rise to enlargement are cystic goitre and exophthalmic goitre. In the former the dilated spaces can be seen on section and the colloid is evidently increased, whilst in the latter the gland is firm and elastic in consistence, and the colloid is scanty. Portions of the tissue should be removed for microscopical examination.

Where there is *diminution* in the size this may be due to a secondary fibrous atrophy or to myxœdema or to cretinism. The gland in such cases may be so small that it may be difficult to find, and may be represented merely by small cysts or small fibrous nodules. More commonly however the reduction in size is less marked and the gland is extremely firm and composed largely of fibrous tissue.

Tumours of the thyroid. These generally are localised to one or other lobe of the gland, though they may be very large, and are most commonly malignant, being either adeno-carcinomatous in type or sarcomatous. Microscopical examination is the only reliable method of differentiating between them.

Accessory thyroids are sometimes found behind the trachea, on the aorta, in the line of the thyro-glossal duct and elsewhere. Glandular structures therefore which are found in these regions should always be cut into and, if any doubt exists as to their nature, should be examined microscopically.

The *parathyroids.* These are ovoid glandular-like bodies found close to the thyroid. Their number varies from four to seven. Usually however four are found, two on each side in close relationship to the postero-lateral aspects of the thyroid, one at least often lying on the posterior surface of the œsophagus or the pharynx.

The *thymus*, the blood vessels and the lymphatic glands have already been examined, but a more complete examination can now be conducted and sections made into the various parts to detect any pathological condition such as tuberculosis, lymphadenoma, etc. If deemed necessary search should now be made for the *sympathetic ganglia.* The superior one which is somewhat fusiform in shape lies close behind the upper part of the internal carotid artery. From this the sympathetic cord is traced downwards to the middle ganglion which lies about the level of the sixth cervical vertebræ. The inferior ganglion is generally attached to the neck of the first rib, and in removing the tissues is frequently left in the body. There is usually, however, no difficulty in finding and recognising the ganglion.

The remaining cervical and thoracic structures. These include the jaws, the parotid and deep cervical glands, the cervical and thoracic vertebræ and the thoracic walls.

The *teeth* and *gums* should be examined for caries, suppurative conditions, etc. Tumours or necrotic changes in the jaws, necrosis or erosions in the vertebræ, the presence of curvature of the spine, ankylosis of the vertebral joints, and overgrowths of bone at any point should be looked for and careful descriptions written.

In cases of tumour growth the extent of the invasion of the bones should be carefully recorded.

The thoracic walls should be examined for fractures, tumours, necrosis, etc.

Parotid, submaxillary and the deep cervical glands. Enlargement of these may be due to acute infective conditions, and in such cases any evidence of suppuration should be looked for. Histological and bacteriological examination of any pus or other secretion is essential, for not only may these tissues be attacked by the pyogenetic organisms but they may also be attacked by such specific organisms as *B. tuberculosis, Streptothrix actinomyces,* etc.

Tumours of the parotid are most commonly a mixture of chondroma, myxoma and adenoma. Endotheliomas are said to be common, and sarcomas also occur. Histological examination should always be undertaken before a definite diagnosis is given.

CHAPTER VII

EXAMINATION OF THE PELVIC CONTENTS

THE PELVIC CONTENTS.

A general examination is made of the structures which have been removed from the pelvis in order to detect any evidence of tumour formation or of adhesions between the various organs. Notes are made of the various pathological conditions found and an examination of the separate organs is undertaken.

(1) *The rectum.* The rectum is slit up from the anal orifice along the posterior (dorsal) wall and carefully examined.

The pathological conditions which are most common are ulceration and tumour formation. The ulceration may be simple, syphilitic or malignant in its character and therefore it will be important to determine the induration, the fibrosis or the degree of infiltration which may be present. If ulcers are found, careful examination should be made for communications between the rectum and the other pelvic viscera. Apart from ulceration, inflammatory conditions in the rectum are not of special pathological importance. Tumours may be adenomatous or epitheliomatous in type. Distension of the venous plexuses in the lower part of the rectum (hæmorrhoids) is looked for. Portions of ulcerated patches including the edge and the adjacent healthy intestine and also portions of tumours with, if possible, the apparently healthy intestine close to the edge of the tumour, should be cut out for histological examination.

Tuberculous ulceration is rare in the rectum but many cases of fistula-in-ano appear to be tuberculous in origin.

Parasites should be looked for, *e.g. Oxyuris vermicularis* and the ova of *Bilharzia hæmatobia*.

(2) *The bladder.* The bladder should be opened along the anterior aspect with a probe-pointed bistoury or with a pair of blunt-pointed scissors introduced through the urethra.

The main pathological conditions are :

(a) *Cystitis* which causes a congestion and swelling of the mucous membrane, the congestion being specially marked at the summit of the ridges. There may be a fibrinous or semi-purulent membrane on the surface or necrotic changes may be extremely marked. In such cases the membrane, the necrotic tissue or the contents of the bladder should be examined bacteriologically. In chronic cases there is usually great thickening of the walls.

(b) *Tuberculosis.* This is usually associated either with tuberculosis of the kidney or tuberculosis which has spread from the epididymis and, therefore, in cases where evidence of tuberculous infection is found in the bladder, a careful examination is directed to the ureters and kidneys and to the prostate, the vas deferens, the seminal vesicles and the epididymis.

(c) *Diverticula* of the bladder should be examined for calculi, and dilatation and hypertrophy noted and an examination made for any causal condition.

(d) *Tumours.* The most common type are the villous papillomata. These may be simple or malignant but by histological examination alone can this be determined ; and therefore portions of the tumour and the wall of the bladder from which the tumour is growing should be cut out and put in fixing solution. Squamous and columnar-celled carcinomas occur but are rare.

(e) The *openings of the ureters* should always be examined for patency.

(f) *Congenital abnormalities.* The various degrees of urinary fistula leading up to complete extroversion of the bladder will have been observed on external examination of the body. In such cases, careful examination must be made for any associated malformations of the urethra and the external genitals.

(g) *Hæmorrhage into or from the bladder.* The causes must be sought. The hæmorrhage may be the result of trauma, calculus formation, blood diseases (*e.g.* hæmophilia, scorbutus, etc.), poisoning (*e.g.* with cantharidin), acute cystitis, tuberculous ulceration, new growths and bilharziasis.

(*h*) *Parasites.* The only parasite of importance which affects the bladder is the *Bilharzia hæmatobia*.

FEMALE GENERATIVE ORGANS.

Uterus and vagina. As a general rule the vagina and uterus are opened by an incision made with the scissors or a bistoury, through the anterior vaginal wall along its mesial line and continued from the cervix to the fundus of the uterus. The uterine incision is made preferably with a probe-pointed bistoury introduced through the external os.

The cavities which are thus opened up are examined, especially as to the condition of their mucous membrane and muscular wall. Endometritis may be present and the endometrium be considerably thickened. Fragments of decidual tissue should be looked for in special cases and attention should be directed to the veins for any evidence of thrombosis and to the muscular wall for suppurative foci.

Carcinoma of the cervix or of the vaginal wall may occur ; but carcinoma or sarcoma of the body of the uterus is not common. Tuberculosis of the wall is rare and is detected only after microscopical examination.

Fibroid tumours (myomas) are common and microscopical examination should be made especially of those which shew any sign of softening or degeneration. Red degeneration, myxomatous changes and sarcomatous transformation may take place, and microscopical examination is therefore essential.

The cervix should always be carefully examined for erosions or for ulcerations, and microscopical examination of such areas is of extreme value for the detection of the early stages of malignant disease. Again microscopical examination of thickened patches or of suspicious areas of new growth in the endometrium is of considerable importance in the recognition of decidual remnants, hydatid mole or chorion epithelioma.

Any abnormalities of the uterus or vagina such as prolapse,

inversion, duplication of cornua, etc. should of course be recorded.

Fallopian tubes. The external examination usually indicates the presence of pathological conditions, and more detailed investigation is made by slitting open the tube in its long axis or by cutting it across transversely to the long axis. The adoption of one or other method will depend on the conditions found.

The most important lesions are salpingitis, tumour formation and tubal gestation.

In cases of salpingitis, especially where the tube is distended and contains purulent material, bacteriological examination should be made, though in many cases the contents are found to be sterile. There seems little doubt that the gonococcus is a common causal organism and in all such cases it should be carefully searched for. Tuberculous salpingitis may sometimes be detected by naked eye examination but the histological examination of a section of the tube is the only certain method of determining definitely the nature of the lesion. Tumours are comparatively rare and tubal gestations usually present very little difficulty to the pathologist. In cases where the tube is thickened and where the diagnosis is not clear it is advisable to make a series of sections for microscopical examination, as only in this way are some pathological conditions, *e.g.* the so-called adeno-myoma, made evident.

Ovaries. External examination will usually be sufficient to detect the important pathological changes, such as cysts and cyst adenomas, dermoid cysts, and tumours. Sections of these cysts or tumours will give further information as to their characters, and microscopical examination will usually clear up any doubt in the diagnosis. Other conditions such as cystic change, fibrosis and calcification in the corpora lutea, abscesses and tuberculosis can hardly fail to be detected, and if doubt occurs a microscopical examination should be undertaken.

The external organs of generation. At this stage, it is convenient to examine the external organs of generation. Pathological changes here are usually so obvious that it is not necessary to do more than enumerate them. Hypertrophy and more rarely atrophy of the vulva, condylomata, gangrenous ulceration in children, abscess of Bartholin's gland, acute inflammatory changes of gonorrhœa, hæmatomas and hernia may be found.

MALE GENERATIVE ORGANS.

The external organs of generation in the male. These are not commonly examined minutely unless there is some special reason to suspect pathological changes in them, but in all cases an external examination of the penis for purulent exudate in the urethra and for evidences of recent or old standing ulceration about the glans should be made. The scrotum and testes should also be examined by inspection and palpation for hernia, hydrocele and tumour formation. Strictures in the urethra should be searched for by means of a catheter.

If it is desired to remove the penis and testicles, the skin should be first carefully dissected from the pubic arch and the inguinal canals opened up. The spermatic cords are isolated and with the forefinger and thumb the testicles are each in turn pushed up out of the scrotum. A few cuts with the knife free them from their attachments. The penis can also be easily shelled out from its covering and cut across about the region of the corona. It is always well to leave the glans and its attachments.

(If it is desired to remove the penis with the bladder and other pelvic organs, the pubic arch should be divided with the saw about one inch on either side of the symphysis, the penis dissected out of the skin covering it and from the surrounding tissues.)

External examination will have revealed the presence of phimosis, of chancres, of condylomata, of gangrenous changes, of soft sores and of malignant growths (epithelioma), and the only point of importance on which more information may be required is the presence, the situation and the nature of strictures. This information may be obtained by slitting up the urethra throughout its whole length. Films and cultures may be made, if thought necessary, for the examination of ulcerated areas, pus, chancres, condylomata, etc.

The epididymis and testis. Sections made into these organs after their removal may give evidence of abscess formation, of tuberculosis, of syphilis and of tumours. In cases of abscess formation or acute inflammatory changes without suppuration, bacteriological examination should be made. In tuberculosis the caseation is usually most marked in, and may be confined to, the epididymis.

In syphilis there may be a dense fibrosis in the testicular tissue or yellowish, caseous gummata are found. Tumours are not common but sarcomas, carcinomas, chorion-epitheliomas and some forms of simple tumours may be found.

Histological examination must always be carried out before a definite diagnosis is given.

Prostate. The most usual pathological condition is hypertrophy and the enlargement is usually most pronounced in the so-called " middle " lobe. Microscopical examination should be made to determine whether the hyperplasia is of the fibrous and muscular tissues or of the glandular part of the organ. Malignant tumours are sometimes with difficulty differentiated from simple hypertrophy and microscopical examination is, of course, essential in such cases. Carcinomata are much more common than sarcomata. Abscesses, tuberculosis and concretions in the prostate should always be looked for and where pus is found bacteriological investigation must be carried out.

CHAPTER VIII

LYMPHATIC GLANDS AND BONE MARROW

LYMPHATIC GLANDS.

The glands which should be specially examined are the cervical, mediastinal, bronchial, mesenteric, axillary and femoral. Palpation or inspection is often sufficient to determine that there is no important pathological lesion in them, but, if there is any doubt, the gland should be cut into, and, where necessary, a histological examination made. The nature of the disease from which the patient has suffered may indicate to the pathologist that special glands should be carefully examined by histological methods. Thus in cancer of the mamma it may be important to examine for any trace of secondary invasion in the axillary glands, again, in cases of tuberculosis of the intestine, the mesenteric glands would be specially examined.

The most important disease conditions in the glands may be briefly summarised as a guide to the pathologist.

Tuberculosis. This is generally quite evident when caseation has taken place, but, in the early stages of the disease only a microscopical examination can determine its presence and in many cases it is of importance to make the examination. In tuberculosis of the cervical glands, the infection often reaches them by way of the tonsils, and therefore it is important to carefully examine these as well as the pharyngeal adenoid tissue.

The bronchial glands may be infected by spread from the cervical glands or by direct spread from the bronchi.

The mesenteric glands are affected by way of the intestine, though no evidence of tuberculosis may be found in the intestine itself.

Lymphadenoma. The glands are affected in association with the spleen and usually the pathologist can have no doubt of the condition except that he may consider the glands to be tuberculous. Microscopical examination in these cases is essential and the presence of tubercle follicles does not exclude the possibility of the case being lymphadenomatous, for tuberculosis is frequently a secondary complication of lymphadenoma. The clinical history of the case and the histological findings usually leave no doubt as to the diagnosis.

Leucocythæmia. The glandular enlargement may be considerable, but the clinical history combined with the examination of the blood, should preclude any possibility of an error in diagnosis.

Acute inflammatory conditions, suppuration and *necrosis* may occur and in these the diagnosis is usually quite obvious. Bacteriological examination should be made in all such cases.

Fibrosis of the glands is common in tuberculosis, in syphilis, and is specially prominent in cases where there has been inhalation of irritating dust over long periods, *e.g.* in quarry workers, in stone cutters and in grinders. This fibrosis is usually associated with pigmentation by carbon.

Amyloid degeneration sometimes occurs in glands, but is usually associated with amyloid changes in such organs as the liver, spleen and kidney, and therefore from a practical point of view is of little importance.

Tumours may be primary as in lymphomas and lympho-sarcomas of the mediastinal glands or more commonly secondary to cancers in various parts of the body. The secondary invasion may often be quite evident to the naked eye, but histological examination is always desirable.

Animal parasites may be found in the glands, *e.g.* hydatids and filariæ.

BONE MARROW.

To examine the bone marrow it is best to remove a few inches of the upper half of the shaft of the femur, though the bone marrow from the ribs may be used; but more reliable information on pathological changes is obtained from the marrow of the long bones.

To obtain marrow from the ribs. The rib is isolated and cut through with bone forceps about 3 or 4 inches posterior to the costo-chondral articulation. By gentle pressure with the forceps, the marrow can be squeezed out from the cut end of the rib on to a glass slide or a small piece of paper. Films are made and preferably fixed, while wet, for a few minutes in a saturated solution of corrosive sublimate or other fixative (Appendix), or the whole mass which has been squeezed out may be fixed in the saturated solution of corrosive sublimate and later sections made of it.

To obtain marrow from the long bones. The femur, as has already been indicated, is chosen and an incision is made on the inner side of the thigh through the skin and subcutaneous tissues and between the muscles from the neck of the bone to the upper limit of the condyles. The bone is thus exposed and it is cut across with a saw about its midpoint. The muscles and other attachments are cut away from the upper half and by very slight manipulation the upper part of the bone is delivered from its bed. It is then cut across just below the trochanter minor. Films should be made from the exposed marrow at the lower end of the isolated portion of bone, or a portion of the marrow should be scooped out from the upper end of the lower portion of the shaft remaining in the body and from this, after fixation, sections can be made.

The portion of bone which has been removed should be split longitudinally, so that the marrow may be examined throughout several inches of the shaft. This is best done by making saw-cuts on the inner and outer side of the shaft from one end to the other but not extending into the medullary canal, and then with a broad chisel, placed across one end of the bone from saw-cut to saw-cut, splitting the bone longitudinally. By this method a neat division is easily made and there is no contamination of the marrow with bone dust from the saw.

(The loss of the portion of bone is replaced by a rounded piece of wood which projects into a hollow scooped out in the upper portion of the bone and into the medullary cavity below.)

For diagnosis of marrow conditions microscopical examinations are essential but the naked eye appearances may give much information.

The healthy marrow in the long bones is " yellow " except at the upper end. When a reaction is taking place changes in colour and in consistence become evident.

The *leucoblastic* marrow which is specially associated with an increase of the leucocytes and is associated with acute infective diseases and acute toxæmias, shews all stages of transference from yellow to red. At first a pinkish colour is seen at the periphery of the shaft and this gradually spreads inwards till the whole of the marrow becomes " pink." Later, if the toxic condition is not arrested, the marrow becomes exhausted and assumes a brownish, translucent or gelatinous appearance and the bony canal becomes widened.

In *leucocythæmia*, the leucoblastic reaction may be extreme and the whole marrow may assume a greyish-pink or even a yellowish-grey colour. In the lymphatic form there may be, in addition, whitish nodules, resembling tumour masses, scattered in various parts.

In the *erythroblastic* condition, the marrow becomes red or even brownish from the deposition of pigment. It may become very soft and the bony trabeculæ of the medullary region may be completely absorbed. This condition is specially seen in severe forms of anæmia, *e.g.* pernicious anæmia and after large hæmorrhages.

Very often in old people the marrow assumes a somewhat greyish, translucent appearance due to gelatinous degeneration, and in such cases there is no apparent reaction as the result of the absorptions of poisons in infective fevers, toxæmias, etc. Secondary deposits of malignant growths are not uncommon in the marrow.

CHAPTER IX

DISEASES OF BONES, JOINTS AND MUSCLES

Bones. The methods to be employed in examining bones must depend on the special condition under examination and the operator must adopt the most suitable plan for investigating and demonstrating the disease or deformity for which he is searching. The most efficacious procedure will usually be to completely dissect out the diseased bone and then section it in various ways. In many cases, however, it will be found that an incision into the bone with a knife or a chisel and the removal of a small portion will be sufficient. The conditions which most commonly call for examination are acute inflammation, chronic abscess, tuberculosis and tumour formation. Where pus is present, bacteriological examination should be undertaken, and microscopical examination made of tumours.

Such diseases as rickets, syphilis, osteomalacia, acromegaly, leontiasis ossea, achondroplasia, etc. may demand special and extensive examination of bones, but for the special characters of these diseases reference should be made to books on special pathology.

Joints. Any incision which will expose the joints thoroughly can be used and the most suitable procedure in any given case must be left to the discretion of the operator. For *bacteriological examination* of joints, the skin and subcutaneous tissues should first be reflected and the deeper tissues seared before the final opening is made into the joint cavity, and this opening must be made with a sterile knife. Not only should the exudate be examined but portions of the synovial membranes, taken at various points, should also be removed for bacteriological examination. I have found that in cases of rheumatism the exudate is usually sterile, whereas streptococci are found in the synovial membranes. In suppurative arthritis, the organisms are usually found in the exudate, but the synovial membrane should also be examined.

All the important diseases of joints are very obvious as soon as the cavity is opened up. Careful descriptions should be written of the conditions found in the tissues round the joints, in the ligaments, in the synovial membranes and in the bone itself.

Muscles. Under exceptional circumstances these require to be carefully examined macroscopically and microscopically but no special method need be described. The pathological conditions which should be looked for are degenerations, atrophy, inflammation and suppuration, tuberculosis, gummata, parasites and tumours.

CHAPTER X

THE CENTRAL NERVOUS SYSTEM

Where it is necessary or desirable to examine the central nervous system carefully the spinal cord should be removed before the brain. By adopting this plan, the operator is enabled to cut through the cord at its upper end cleanly and quite transversely and the upper part of the cord is removed with the brain at a later stage of the examination.

Removal of spinal cord. The body is placed face downwards, with the head hanging over the end of the table. The
natural curves of the spinal column are got rid of as far as
possible by placing blocks under the body particularly in the
dorso-lumbar region. Standing at the head of the body the
operator, with his left hand placed over the sacral region,
puts the skin on the stretch, and then plunges his cartilage
knife through the skin, the subcutaneous tissues and the
muscle down to the sacrum slightly to the left of the middle
line. The knife, which is now at an angle of about 60° with
the skin surface above it, is drawn firmly upward through all
the tissues lying between the skin surface and the bone, from
the sacrum to the occiput—the skin meanwhile being kept on
the stretch with the left hand.

This incision will lie immediately to the left of the spinous
processes and its floor will be the laminæ of the vertebræ.
A similar incision is now made on the right side through the
muscular tissue from which the skin has been retracted.

With a moderately heavy saw, such as the common full-
bladed one used by butchers, the laminæ are completely sawn
through just internal to the articular processes. This line of
incision is very important, for if the cut is made too near the
middle line there is great difficulty in freeing and extracting
the cord, whereas, if it is too far out, the roof of the canal is
difficult to remove. In the lumbar region the articular processes are easily detected, and in the cervical the line of the
saw cut is indicated by a shallow groove at the outer extremity
of the laminæ. If the saw is placed in this groove and immediately internal to the lumbar articular processes, the line of
incision is definitely indicated. It will be seen that the saw-
cut inclines slightly outwards as it passes from cervical to
lumbar region. It is often found more convenient to complete
the cervical saw-cut in the reverse direction, *i.e.* sawing from
below upwards. Corresponding incisions are made on either
side of the spinal processes. Only in the dorsal region is there
danger of damaging the cord by cutting completely through
the laminæ and, with ordinary care, this danger should be
avoided.

It is generally necessary to divide the upper cervical laminæ with bone forceps. Having now completed the incisions the interspinous ligaments and the ligamenta flava are divided between two vertebræ in the mid-dorsal region with the bone forceps. Either with the hand or with lion forceps, the upper dorsal spinous processes are seized, and if the saw-cut has been properly made, the whole posterior wall of the upper part of the vertebral column can be pulled away without any difficulty. If, however, the laminæ have not been sawn completely it may be necessary to complete the separation with bone forceps, pulling up the spinous processses and laminæ with lion forceps and cutting first on one side and then on the other with the bone forceps.

The lower portion of the spinal cord is laid bare in a similar manner and any projecting spicules of bone removed with the bone forceps.

Before the cord is removed from the spinal canal note should be made of any pathological conditions which have been found such as hæmorrhages into the muscles resulting from bruises, tumours invading the muscle or projecting into the canal, abnormalities in the bones, fractures, caries, etc. and any evidence of purulent infiltration, particularly into the loose fatty tissue which is found in the dorsal aspect of the spinal canal. This fatty tissue should be removed so that the cord may be fully exposed, for inspection of the cord may give evidence of purulent collections resulting from meningitis, of softening of tumours, etc. and, if such conditions are suspected, it may be necessary to modify the method of examination. Usually, however, the next procedure is to pass a sharp bistoury downwards along each lateral aspect of the dura mater, so as to divide the nerve roots. A fold of the dura mater at its lower end is now pinched up with dissecting forceps and it, together with the cauda equina, is cut completely across with a sharp-curved bistoury.

The cord is now raised out of the canal and, while extending it with the left hand, and cutting through the loose cellular tissue between the dura and the posterior common ligament, it is completely removed from the spinal canal.

Before cutting through the cord at its upper end, which should be done transversely and immediately below the foramen magnum, the connective tissue which attaches the dura to the posterior common ligament in this situation should be divided completely.

If special examination of the spinal ganglia is required, *e.g.* in cases of ascending and descending degenerations in the cord, the transverse processes of the vertebræ are removed with bone forceps and the ganglia dissected out from the intervertebral foramina, in the preliminary stages of the operation for the removal of the cord, before the nerve roots are cut. It is easier, however, to dissect out the ganglia after the removal of the cord and unless it is necessary to maintain their connections with the cord this procedure is followed.

The methods which have been described above are those which are adopted in the majority of cases, but special conditions may arise, *e.g.* abnormalities in the cord or in the spinal column, which may render these methods inapplicable in all their details, but modifications of methods to suit individual cases must be left to the intelligence of the operator.

After removal, the cord is placed on a flat table, with the posterior surface uppermost, and the dura mater is slit along the middle line posteriorly, care being taken not to puncture the cord with the scissors. The dura may be adherent to the arachnoid at various points, but these adhesions are usually easily separated by pulling on the dura with a pair of dissecting forceps. The cord is then turned over and the membranes on the anterior surface treated in a similar fashion.

During and after these operations note should be made of any adhesions between the dura and the arachnoid, of thickenings of the dura or of the arachnoid, of the presence of bony plates, of subdural pus or blood, of subarachnoid pus and of special thickenings of the pia-arachnoid.

In cases of syphilis and in tuberculosis the pia-arachnoid should be most carefully examined for evidence of syphilitic or tuberculous meningitis.

Further naked eye examination by inspection and by gentle

palpation may reveal areas of softening (myelitis) or areas of greater resistance (sclerosis), may give evidence of tumours, of gummata, of tuberculous nodules and of hæmorrhages, but most of the degenerative and sclerotic diseases of the spinal cord are only with certainty detected on careful histological examination. It is therefore of special importance that the cord should be properly preserved. It is first cut into lengths of 8 to 10 cm. by transverse incisions which are made just below the points of entrance of the posterior nerve roots. The dura is not cut and by threads passed through this membrane the cord is suspended in the fixing fluid. (Appendix.)

Such conditions as spina-bifida, all forms of lepto-meningitis, and acute myelitis are obvious on naked eye examination, but bacteriological examination should always be made in the two latter conditions and histological examination may be of value in myelitis.

The general condition of the vessels of the cord should always be examined for thickening (arterio-sclerosis) and for thrombosis. Though certain naked eye appearances such as local congestion, local adhesions and local atrophy, etc. may be seen in degenerative conditions such as locomotor ataxia, lateral sclerosis, progressive muscular atrophy, amyotrophic lateral sclerosis, poliomyelitis, chronic myelitis and syringomyelia, but little importance can be attached to these from the diagnostic standpoint and therefore histological, and it may be bacteriological, examinations are essential to establish a post-mortem diagnosis.

Examination of the scalp and skull. The body lies on its back and the head is supported on a hollowed-out wooden block placed under the occiput. In females, the hair is parted in a line extending across the vertex of the scalp from mastoid process to mastoid process. An incision is now made through the tissues of the scalp, right to the bone, over the left mastoid process. A knife with a thin blade of medium length is inserted under the tissues of the scalp at this incision—the back of the knife being towards the bone—and carried across the vertex to the mastoid process of the opposite side (Plate VII). Thus the scalp is divided from within outwards, as less destruction of the hair takes place than by cutting from without inwards.

Any tissues which have not been completely divided are now dealt with by means of another incision which extends to the pericranium. The anterior half of the scalp is dissected up and drawn forward over the face until the line of reflexion reaches the upper margins of the orbit. This separation of the scalp is usually very easy of accomplishment if the primary incision has been satisfactorily made. The posterior half is treated in a similar fashion and, when completed, the occipital protuberance should be exposed.

Examination is made of the scalp and of the exposed portion of the skull.

The *scalp* should be examined for hæmorrhages or other evidence of injury, scars, suppuration, and tumours, especially of the cystic type, and the *skull* for the condition of the fontanelles in children, for evidences of fracture, for softened areas (cranio-tabes, syphilis, etc.), for bony tumours (ivory exostoses and Parrot's nodes) and for tumours or gummata which have started primarily on the bone or which have invaded it secondarily. Careful note should be made of any pathological condition which may be found.

Removal of the skull cap. The knife is drawn circumferentially round the skull in the line in which it is intended to make the saw-cut and the expansions of the temporal muscles together with the temporal fascia divided down to the bone in that line.

This line in its anterior aspect is about 1 cm. ($\frac{1}{2}$ inch) above the orbital margins or midway between the highest point of the orbital margins and the frontal eminences and posteriorly it passes through the posterior occipital protuberance.

Having made this line with the knife, the saw-cut follows it exactly in the anterior and lateral aspects of the skull, but, in my opinion, it is better to depart from the line posteriorly in the following manner (Plate VIII).

The lateral saw-cut on each side ends at the point at which this line crosses the lambdoidal suture or slightly anterior to this in the plane of the posterior border of the mastoid process.

Plate VII

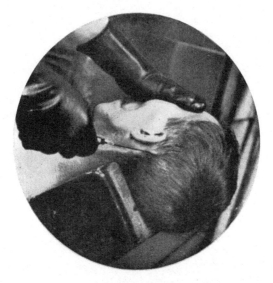

Fig. 11. Shewing position of the knife in the preliminary
stage to incising the scalp.

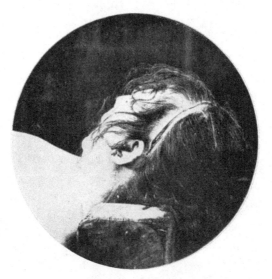

Fig. 12. Shewing the parting of the hair and the
incision through the scalp.

From these points two saw-cuts are now made which meet at
a point above the external occipital protuberance midway
between it and the lambda. The advantage of this method
is that it enables the skull cap to be replaced very accurately
and to be so securely fixed in position that there is no dis-
figurement of the forehead by the slipping back of the skull
cap—an appearance so commonly seen when the common
method of complete circumferential incision is followed. It is
said that by adopting this method there is more likelihood of
damage to the occipital lobes and the cerebellum when the brain
is being removed, but my experience is not in agreement with
this view. With ordinary care, there is no risk of damage.
When sawing through the bone the head should be held very
firmly and I have always found this more conveniently done
by pressing on the vertex with the left hand which is protected
by a towel. If an assistant is available it is a great help to
get him to hold the head steady.

It is not of great importance to completely divide the bone
throughout the whole length of the saw-cut, except in cases
where fracture of the bones is suspected, and in such cases the
greatest care must be taken lest any artificial fracture is brought
about by rough manipulation and therefore the bone must be
completely divided with the saw, even at the risk of damaging
the brain.

The chisel is introduced into the anterior part of the saw-
cut and by rotation of it a sufficient opening is made to introduce the fingers of the left hand, protected by a towel. If there
is difficulty in thus opening up the frontal saw-cut, it may be
found necessary with the chisel and mallet to break at various
points portions of the bone which have not been completely
sawn through. When this has been accomplished gentle pressure will easily separate the calvarium from the rest of the
skull unless there are firm adhesions between it and the dura
mater. These adhesions may be separated with the handle of
a scalpel or with a periosteal elevator ; or, if they are very firm,
the dura is removed with the calvarium. In young children it
is generally advisable to remove the dura with the calvarium
by cutting it through in the line of the saw-cut.

In very young children, those under six months, the skull
cap is so flexible that by merely opening up thoroughly the
fontanelles and sutures and partially cutting the skull with
strong scissors in the usual circumferential line, it may be found
possible to remove the brain without actually removing the
calvarium.

Examination of the calvarium and the exposed dura mater.
Fractures are specially examined and their exact extent and
location determined. Other abnormalities such as necrosis,
tumours, thinning or absorption of bone, thickening of the
skull or dura, gummata or other evidences of syphilis in bone
or dura are carefully noted and exact descriptions of the conditions found are recorded. Where there is evidence of extra-
dural hæmorrhage, careful examination is made of the middle
meningeal artery and its branches. The longitudinal sinus is
now slit up and the condition of the contained blood noted—
especially as to evidence of thrombosis.

The dura is next reflected. It is pinched up on each side
at any point in the frontal region close to the bone, an incision
made through it and then with a probe-pointed bistoury, which
has been introduced through the incision, it is cut from within
outwards along the line of the saw-cut. The attachment of
the falx cerebri to the crista galli is cut with a bistoury passed
inwards in the middle line in front, while the falx is pulled
upwards with dissecting forceps. The whole dural covering
is now drawn backwards and the surface of the brain is
exposed.

Before removal of the brain, note should be made of any
pathological condition observed after stripping the dura, such
as flattening of the convolutions, dryness of the pia, the presence
of congestion or of purulent exudate indicating meningitis and
the presence of hæmorrhage. The flattening of the convolutions and the dryness of the membranes may be general or
localised and indicate distension of one or both lateral ventricles,
hæmorrhage into the substance of the brain, an abscess, a cyst
or a tumour, and therefore may be an important sign of localisation of these pathological conditions. If pus or blood is seen,
the operator should determine whether it is subpial or merely

Plate VIII

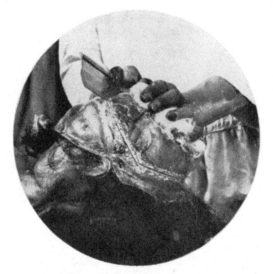

Fig. 13. Shewing method of holding skull during the sawing and on one side the lines of the saw cuts.

subdural. If subdural it can be rubbed or washed off the surface, if subpial it remains till the pia is lacerated.

Tumours, etc. which may be evident at this stage of the operation are better examined after the brain has been removed.

In chronic alcoholics and in the insane the condition of *pachymeningitis hæmorrhagica* should be looked for, and is evidenced by the presence of a reddish-brown, rather firm membranous layer covering the inner surface of the dura. Gummata and tumours of the dura must be borne in mind in making the examination and careful note made of any such condition. Of the tumours, sarcomata are most frequently found, though fibromata and osteomata have been described.

Removal of the brain. The frontal lobes are raised gently out of the anterior fossæ either with the handle of a scalpel or with the fingers of the left hand and the olfactory bulbs are freed from the cribriform plates. The optic nerves and the internal carotid arteries are now divided and the infundibulum is separated from the pituitary body. The brain is allowed to fall backwards by its own weight, the left hand, however, acting as a slight support. The third and the fourth nerves are divided and then with the bistoury the tentorium cerebelli is cut close to the petrous temporal bone. The sixth and the fifth nerves are usually divided while the tentorium is being cut. The other cranial nerves are divided in order and then the vertebral artery is cut. If the spinal cord has been removed in the way already indicated, the brain should now be free and will slip out on to the left hand if the cerebellum is gently raised by the fingers of the right hand placed on its under surface. If the spinal cord has not been removed previous to removal of the brain, the cord is cut across transversely after the vertebral arteries have been divided.

Before proceeding to the examination of the brain, the lateral sinuses, the circular and the straight sinuses should be opened up and examined for any evidence of septic infection or thrombosis. The pituitary body may be removed easily by first chiselling off the posterior clinoid processes and the posterior wall of the sella turcica—a single blow of the chisel is usually sufficient to accomplish this. The pituitary is then easily dissected out of the sella turcica.

Examination of the brain. Unless there are special reasons for examining sections of the brain at once it is advisable, after making careful notes of any obvious pathological changes, to put the whole organ into a fixing solution (5 to 10 % formalin) so as to harden it before further examination is made, and in some cases careful injection with formalin by way of the basal arteries is desirable.

External examination. The brain should be weighed and attention directed to the following points in the external examination :

(1) *Hæmorrhage.* The extent and the exact situation of this should be noted, as these may be important indications as to the site from which the blood has come. Thus a localised area at the base of the brain may suggest a ruptured aneurism in the circle of Willis, extensive subpial hæmorrhage may indicate ruptured pial vessels but more commonly this is the result of a central hæmorrhage which has burst into the lateral ventricle and has passed along the ventricular system to the subarachnoid space, while a mass of blood outside the pia suggests injury or rupture of diseased vessels in the dura or the pia, rupture of an aneurism in the larger cerebral vessels, especially the anterior cerebral, sinus thrombosis, or damage to vessels in injury to the bones of the skull.

Multiple subarachnoid hæmorrhages occur in certain cases of acute infective diseases. of purpura, of scurvy, of leucocythæmia and of pernicious anæmia. Extensive subarachnoid hæmorrhage has been described in cases of anthrax, and therefore it is important in any case in which a cause for the hæmorrhage is not obvious to make a bacteriological examination.

(2) *Meningitis.* In most of the acute cases there is usually no difficulty in diagnosis, the purulent exudate shewing itself under the pia, both at the base and over the vertex. In some cases of tuberculous meningitis and of cerebro-spinal and posterior-basal meningitis the exudate may be scanty and confined to the interpeduncular region. In such cases histological examination of the exudate is essential and, in

non-tuberculous cases, a bacteriological examination should always be made. In tuberculous meningitis there is usually well marked viscid greenish exudate, with thickening of the membranes in the interpeduncular space, and though minute tubercle granulations are present they may be obscured by the exudate. The granulations are usually better seen in the extensions of the pia which pass up the Sylvian fissures and should always be looked for in that situation. They are also sometimes seen on the vertex and in the dura covering the base of the skull.

In posterior-basal meningitis there may be very little turbid exudate and comparatively little thickening of the membranes. In such cases and in all acute forms of meningitis, bacteriological examination should be made to determine the causal organism. Attempts have been made to differentiate the various types of meningitis by a localisation of the purulent exudate, but this, in my opinion, is very likely to lead to erroneous conclusions. The operator, it is true, may form some general idea of the causal organism from naked eye examination, but a bacteriological examination must be regarded as essential to a correct diagnosis.

In some forms of rapidly fatal meningitis there may be little or no exudate, but usually the membranes are dry and sticky. Unless a bacteriological examination is made in such cases the meningitis may be entirely overlooked.

(3) *The Pacchionian bodies.* These must be carefully noted. Normally they are opaque white bodies projecting from the arachnoid, and are situated along the margins of the great longitudinal fissure. They may penetrate the dura and erode the bones of the skull. Sometimes they are poorly developed and, by the inexperienced, have been mistaken for tubercle granulations. Their localisation should be sufficient to prevent such an error.

(4) *Chronic thickenings of the membranes* are seen in alcoholic subjects and are also associated with syphilis. In the latter condition the thickening may be accompanied by small miliary gummata or even with larger gummatous masses which are most commonly found at the base of the brain, causing pressure on one or more of the cranial nerves.

(5) *The convolutions.* Note should be made of any flattening or narrowing of the convolutions with corresponding changes in the sulci. Localised atrophy, congenital abnormalities and the results of injury should be looked for. In general atrophy the convolutions are narrowed and the sulci deepened, the membranes are thickened and the weight of the brain as a whole is lessened.

(6) *Œdema.* This is a very common condition and it may be the only lesion found in cases where the symptoms pointed to cerebral hæmorrhage or to tumour formation. The condition is best appreciated before the brain is removed from the skull, the œdematous fluid filling up the sulci and often presenting a somewhat gelatinous appearance. On section of the brain the white matter is usually softened and extremely moist.

(7) *The vessels.* These should be examined for any sign of arterio-sclerosis or aneurism, and special attention directed to those at the base of the brain.

Further examination of the brain (before or after hardening in a fixative). The cerebellum and pons are separated from the cerebrum either by dividing the crura cerebri just above the pons or by dividing the pons transversely just above the roots of the fifth cranial nerves. In most cases the first method is followed, but if for any reason it is specially important to examine the third nerve the second method must be used, for, in cutting through the crura cerebri the third nerve is likely to be damaged.

The cerebellum, pons and medulla are now examined : one or two cuts, extending almost through its substance and parallel with its surface are made in the cerebellum and various transverse sections are made in the pons and the medulla. Evidence of hæmorrhage, of softening, of tumour formation, of tuberculosis in the form of tuberculous masses and of gummata can hardly be missed if these incisions are made. Degenerative changes in the conducting areas may also be apparent in the transverse sections, but histological examination should always be made in order to confirm the naked eye appearances.

The cerebrum. It is hardly advisable to lay down definite rules for examination of the cerebrum for a common method is not applicable. The condition which is suspected or the condition which, from external examination, the operator knows he will find, will determine in any given case how the brain should be cut. The essential point is that the brain should be cut in such a way that the best exposure is made of the pathological lesions.

In the majority of cases, I have found the old method of making several complete sections of the brain, parallel to its long axis, quite satisfactory. The sections should not be too thick—the *third* should pass through the upper part of the basal ganglia and open up the lateral ventricles. If further examination is needed, for example for areas of softening, a series of sections, transverse to the long axis, are made from the frontal region to the occiput through the various horizontal sections which have already been made.

Most of the gross pathological lesions of the substance of the brain are easily recognised on naked eye examination and, though indications may also be given of the finer degenerative changes, only histological examination is satisfactory in the determination of these.

Cerebral hæmorrhage. If this condition is found, its exact position and its extent should be described ; and in particular its relation to the basal ganglia and the lateral ventricles determined. Search should be made for the causal condition, attention being specially directed to the vessels for signs of arterio-sclerosis and for aneurism. It must always be borne in mind that hæmorrhages may occur in association with tumours (sarcomata and gliomata), in scurvy and in purpura and in certain blood-diseases such as leucocythæmia and pernicious anæmia.

Examination should be made for any evidences of old hæmorrhages. They are usually indicated by irregular cyst-like spaces, the walls of which are yellowish from altered blood pigment. Fluid is sometimes present and in some cases hæmosiderin granules and hæmatoidin crystals may be demonstrated.

Cerebral softening. The areas may vary considerably in size, but are usually easily detected by their semi-fluid consistence in the fresh condition, and in the hardened brain they are usually distinctly mapped out from the normal tissue. Microscopical examination shews necrosis and loss of definite structure in the various nerve elements of the area. Search must always be made for the causal condition, particularly for thrombosis or embolism. The site of the softened area will indicate to the operator the probable vessel. Thrombosis is more common in the cortical vessels and is usually secondary to degenerative conditions in their walls. Embolism occurs more often on the left side and in the central vessels and is commonly associated with cardiac disease—vegetations on the valves or thrombosis in some of the chambers. Softening may also be found round tumours and associated with acute inflammatory changes (*acute encephalitis*). In the latter condition there are usually minute hæmorrhages in the centrum ovale, in the basal ganglia and sometimes in the cerebellum and pons. Old softened patches are usually represented by cyst-like spaces containing clear fluid, and the walls are not usually stained unless there has been associated hæmorrhage.

Abscesses (*acute suppurative encephalitis*). This condition is usually secondary to disease of the cranial bones or disease of the middle ear and these pathological conditions always suggest to the operator a careful examination of the brain for suppuration, and on the other hand abscesses in the brain should always lead to an examination for some primary focus. Metastatic suppuration is usually seen under or in the cortex near the vertex, or in the tempero-sphenoidal lobe and may be secondary to empyema, septic pneumonia, chronic lung disease with dilatation and suppuration in the bronchi, infective endocarditis, actinomycosis and wounds of the bones, etc. Round the abscess there is always an area of softening in the early stages, but later there may be formed a definite wall of granulation tissue. Bacteriological examination should be made in all these cases.

Chronic encephalitis (*sclerosis*). Greyish or greyish-red patches may be found in various positions in the white matter, but satisfactory demonstration of such areas can only be made with the aid of the microscope.

Hydrocephalus. A slight degree of dilatation of the lateral ventricles is not uncommon and no obvious cause may be found. In other cases the dilatation is associated with meningitis and is due to the closure of the foramen of Majendie and the lateral recesses of the fourth ventricle. A similar condition may arise by pressure of tumours on the veins of Galen or by closure of the aqueduct of Sylvius by tumours about the fourth ventricle, cerebellum or pons. In congenital hydrocephalus the cause is seldom evident, but in some cases intrauterine meningitis may be the cause of the dilatation.

Tumours of the brain. These can hardly be missed by a careful operator and an accurate diagnosis can only be made after microscopical examination. The position of the tumour should be very accurately recorded and particularly its relation to the nerves, nerve roots, nerve nuclei and other important structures. The size of the tumour and its general naked eye characters should be noted.

The more common cerebral tumours are gliomata, and sarcomas, but psammomas, epitheliomas, teratomas, cholesteatomas and columnar-celled carcinomas may occur. Such tumours must be distinguished from gummata and from tuberculous masses.

The pituitary body. The method of removal has already been noted and the main conditions to be looked for are enlargement and tumour formation.

The peripheral nerves. Only under special circumstances are these examined and the nature of the case must determine the special nerve and the portion of it which should be examined. Tumours are easily detected but their nature must be determined with the microscope as must any evidence of degeneration and regeneration.

CHAPTER XI

POST-MORTEM EXAMINATION FOR
MEDICO-LEGAL PURPOSES

External examination. If the preliminary examination is
made where the body is found careful notes should be taken of
the position in which it was lying, the general appearance of
the face, the position of the arms and hands and, if the hands
are clenched, any substances grasped by them should be examined. The fingers should be carefully looked at for cuts,
or bruises, and scratches or cuts about the face should be noted.
The condition of the dress and any obvious stains upon it may
be of special importance. The condition of the ground around
the body should be examined for signs of a struggle and for
objects which may have been dropped by the victim or by
the assailant. The temperature of the body and any signs of
rigidity or of putrefaction should be noted. The results of
this preliminary examination should be at once recorded in
writing.

After the body has been removed to the mortuary or other
convenient place, the clothes are taken off and any wounds
are carefully compared in position with tears, cuts, etc. in the
clothing. Bruises should be examined and their exact situation
and size recorded. Surface markings, and abnormalities or
pathological changes which may be useful for identification
should be noted—such as pigmentation areas, tattoo marks,
scars of wounds or of diseased conditions, nævi or other " birth
marks," natural or acquired abnormalities about the fingers
or the toes, the condition of the teeth, the colour of the hair,
height, weight, muscular development, sex, age, etc. In women
and children the presence or absence of the hymen, any signs
of recent violence to the genital organs, the presence or absence
of striæ gravidarum and the presence of foreign bodies in any
of the natural passages should be ascertained.

All wounds should be examined carefully to ascertain their
exact extent and position, and their characteristics especially as

to whether they could have been self-inflicted and what sort of instrument might have been employed. Finger marks, especially about the neck, and signs of strangulation should be looked for. If there is evidence of a gunshot wound, the tissues round it should be carefully examined for blackening, etc.

Internal examination. The methods to be followed are those described in previous chapters. A complete examination must be made in every case, even though sufficient cause of death is found on a preliminary examination. The cavity supposed to be implicated should be opened first, and in examining the brain it is of the greatest importance, if any injury to the bone is suspected, that the saw alone should be used in removing the calvarium. All penetrating wounds should be carefully examined and their direction, site and general characters specially noted in order to determine if possible whether they have been self-inflicted or not. The vagina and the uterus should be carefully examined for signs of recent delivery and for mechanical injuries. The condition of the stomach, *e.g.* whether it is empty or whether it contains undigested or partially digested food, may be of the greatest importance in helping to determine the period at which death took place

Cases of Suspected Poisoning.

The history of the case should, if possible, be ascertained and especially the time which has elapsed between the death and the post-mortem examination. The presence or absence of rigor mortis and the extent and general characters of any lividity which may be present may be of considerable importance. Bruises, hæmorrhages or other signs of violence and the nature (colour and general characteristics) of any stains or evidence of necrosis on any part of the body, but especially about the lips, should be carefully described. Where the poison has been taken by the mouth it is essential that the whole of the alimentary tract should be carefully examined and that the contents should be carefully collected in thoroughly clean glass vessels.

The mouth and lips should be examined for injuries caused by corrosives.

In the *abdomen* the points which call for special attention are evidences of peritonitis, especially on the peritoneal aspect of the stomach, perforation or other necrotic changes in the alimentary tract, and any special pathological changes such as fatty condition or necrosis in the various viscera. If any of the contents have escaped from the alimentary canal these should be carefully collected in a perfectly clean glass vessel. Any unusual odour should receive attention. The condition of the blood in the various vessels—its colour and its consistence—should be noted.

In the *thorax* attention is directed to the condition of the œsophagus, to the colour of the lungs and to the condition of the blood in the heart—the cavities being opened up for this purpose. Some of the blood should be collected in a special vessel.

In the *cervical* tissues any evidences of necrosis or staining should be looked for.

Double ligatures should now be placed round the œsophagus immediately below the diaphragm, on the jejunum close to its commencement, on the small intestine just above the ileo-cœcal valve, and on the rectum as far down in the pelvis as possible.

The cervical tissues with the tongue, tonsils and pharynx are dissected out in the manner described and these, together with the thoracic organs including the aorta, the œsophagus, the thoracic duct and portions of the diaphragm are removed *en masse*—the œsophagus having been divided below the diaphragm between the two ligatures which have been previously applied, and the aorta and other structures being cut across above the diaphragm. Great care should be taken in manipulating the tissues, especially in cases where necrotic changes have been produced by the action of corrosive poisons.

The *small intestines* are next removed in the ordinary way (p. 40), having been divided between the ligatures at the jejunal origin and above the ileo-cœcal valve. The *large intestine* is then removed, special care being taken not to injure the duodenum when removing the upper part of the ascending and the transverse colon.

The remaining parts of the *œsophagus*, the *stomach*, the *duodenum*, the *liver*, the *spleen*, the *suprarenals* and the *pancreas* are removed *en masse*, special care being taken that the stomach is not damaged.

The kidneys, in continuity with the ureters and bladder, are next removed in association with the other pelvic contents (p. 42).

Eexamination of the Tissues and Organs which have been removed.

Cervical and thoracic. The pharynx and œsophagus are slit up along the mesial line posteriorly and their mucous membrane carefully examined, along with the tongue, the epiglottis and the tonsils, for evidence of necrosis, of corrosion or of staining. The trachea is opened and the incision continued well into the intrapulmonary bronchi, so that the lining membrane of these passages may be carefully examined. The heart, which has been previously opened, is separated from the lungs, and the valves, etc. examined in the manner described on p. 45. The heart, the lungs and the rest of the cervical and thoracic tissues are put into clean vessels in case chemical examination may be deemed necessary.

The stomach, duodenum, liver, etc. The contents of the stomach and duodenum, and those of the gall bladder are collected in separate vessels and then the œsophagus, the stomach and the duodenum are opened and carefully examined for staining, for congestion, for ulceration and for necrosis. Search should be made with the aid of a lens for crystals of poisons, fragments of leaves, berries, other parts of plants, etc.

Care must be taken to differentiate between necrosis and post-mortem digestion of the stomach. The liver, the spleen, the suprarenals and the pancreas are examined in the ordinary way and the whole of the organs placed in clean jars in case they should be needed for subsequent chemical examination.

The intestines are next examined, the contents of the small and of the large intestine collected in separate vessels and careful inspection made of the mucous membrane for any pathological changes.

The *kidneys* and the *pelvic viscera* are examined in the usual way and the organs kept in clean jars in case they should be needed for chemical examination. The urine should be collected in a separate vessel.

The central nervous system. The examination is conducted in the ordinary way, and the brain and spinal cord kept in separate vessels for further examination.

All jars or other vessels in which the organs or the contents of heart, alimentary canal, etc. are kept should be closed, carefully labelled and sealed immediately after the examination. The labels should give a description of the contents, the name of the individual, and the date of the post-mortem examination.

Corrosive Poisons.

Sulphuric acid, hydrochloric acid, and *nitric acid.* The changes produced by these acids are very similar in their general characters and the differences between the appearances are comparatively unimportant. With *hydrochloric acid* there may be no visible alteration about the lips, whereas with *sulphuric* or *nitric acid* the lips and sometimes the surrounding skin shew marked yellowish or brownish corroded areas. Again, the mucous membrane of the stomach often shews a greenish-yellow discolouration, though dark brown or even black patches are commonly present in cases of poisoning with *nitric acid,* whereas in poisoning by *sulphuric* or *hydrochloric acid* the mucous membrane becomes dark brown or black.

Perforation of the stomach is common in poisoning with *sulphuric acid* but rare where *hydrochloric* or *nitric acid* is the agent used. With all three the mucous membrane of the mouth and pharynx may be greyish-white, brownish-yellow or dark brown in colour, dry and extensively corroded or necrosed. The tissues lying under the membrane are swollen and congested.

In the œsophagus similar changes may be seen and in the stomach there may be very extensive softening and separation of the mucous membrane or irregular erosions of varying size.

The stomach usually shews these changes in a more marked degree than the œsophagus. It is usually contracted and the mucous membrane may be largely destroyed or it may be corrugated and hardened. The staining has already been noted. The inflammation may be so intense that all the coats are disorganised, and, this condition, which will lead to perforation, is most common in cases where *sulphuric acid* has been the poisoning agent. Similar though less marked changes may be found in the intestines.

The other organs shew no specially characteristic naked eye changes, though microscopically there may be necrosis and fatty changes in the cells of the liver and the kidney.

If the patient lives for some weeks, evidence of ulceration, cicatrisation and contraction, producing definite strictures, may be found.

Oxalic acid and *acetic acid.* The changes may be similar to those seen in hydrochloric acid poisoning if a strong solution of acid is swallowed, but if a weak solution has been used the signs are principally those of congestion and inflammation (irritant poisoning). The lips are not stained or corroded, the mucous membrane of the mouth, pharynx and œsophagus is whitened and eroded, and that of the stomach is pale at places, softened and often extensively eroded. There may be irregular dark patches similar to those seen in cases of poisoning by sulphuric acid and due to alterations in the blood. Perforation is rare. The degree of erosion varies greatly in different cases.

The stomach usually contains a dark brown, mucous fluid of a very acid reaction. Calcium oxalate may be very abundant in the kidneys, and may appear as a distinct white line between the cortex and the medulla in cases in which oxalic acid has been swallowed.

Potassium binoxalate (salts of sorrel or salts of lemon) produces similar changes to those seen in oxalic acid poisoning and, in both cases, punctiform hæmorrhages are often seen in the folds of the mucous membrane in the stomach and also in the intestine. In some cases, bleeding from the intestine is a marked feature of the condition.

Alkalies. Ammonia, caustic potash and *caustic soda.* In

ammonia poisoning the effects of the vapour are sometimes marked in the larynx where the mucous membrane may become congested, infiltrated and covered with a false membrane. These conditions become exaggerated if the liquid ammonia comes in contact with the mucous membrane.

With all the *alkalies* there is congestion and swelling of the mucous membrane of the mouth, pharynx, œsophagus, stomach, and sometimes of the duodenum. There may be numerous erosions or larger ulcers. The softening and necrosis with partial separation of the membrane is usually a well marked feature. The deeper tissues are inflamed and congested. The colour varies with the different alkalies. With *ammonia* the surface becomes stained a yellowish colour and with *caustic potash* and *caustic soda* a deep brown or black.

The contents of the stomach are turbid, usually bloodstained, and frequently coffee-coloured. The muscular wall of the œsophagus and stomach may be softened and degenerated and perforation may occur, especially in cases of poisoning with ammonia.

The other organs do not shew any very characteristic changes, the liver may be fatty, the spleen enlarged and congested, and the kidney may shew extensive degeneration of the cells of the secreting tubules. If the patient survives some time, broncho-pneumonia may develop, especially in cases of ammonia poisoning, where the larynx is affected and, at later stages, scars and cicatricial contraction may be found.

IRRITANT POISONS.

Arsenic. Decomposition is usually retarded, sometimes for many months. In the acute cases this retardation may not be appreciable.

Acute poisoning. There is intense local irritation and inflammation in the stomach and the intestines, the mucous membrane being covered with mucus or even with purulent lymph. Hæmorrhages are common and the mucous membrane may be intensely red and at parts gangrenous. Perforation does not occur and well formed ulcers are rarely seen.

The œsophagus usually escapes, but the stomach and, to a less extent, the duodenum and other parts of the intestine shew the changes described above. The solitary glands and Peyer's patches are often swollen. There is in addition acute degenerative changes in the secreting cells of the kidney with fatty degeneration in the liver, the heart and the endothelium of the blood vessels. Where much vomiting has taken place, patches of corrosion may be found in the mouth and on the lips. Particles of the poison are sometimes found entangled in the mucus in the stomach or embedded near the erosions.

The more profound changes are produced by the local action of the arsenic, but even when arsenic has entered the system by some other channel than the mouth, the gastritis may still be well developed.

In exceptional cases paralysis of the nerve centres may be the main symptom, and, on post-mortem examination, the amount of gastro-enteritis may be extremely small, in spite of the fact that large quantities of arsenic may be found in the stomach.

Chronic poisoning. There is distinct evidence of wasting of the tissues, suggesting malnutrition and the skin is pigmented (yellowish-brown or brownish-black), and not uncommonly shews eczematous eruptions. The exposed parts may be ulcerated and in one case which I saw there was definite evidence of secondary epitheliomatous change. The stomach shews a varying degree of inflammatory changes, sometimes with ulceration or even gangrene. Its mucous membrane is covered with tenacious mucus which may be blood-stained. The cardiac end of the stomach shews the changes more markedly than the pyloric end, and, in some cases, definite evidence of a deposit of arsenious acid is found in the inflamed areas. The duodenum, the jejunum, the ascending colon and the rectum may shew changes similar to those found in the stomach, and the small intestine may give evidence of inflammation with swelling of the Peyer's patches and multiple minute ulcers. Fatty and other degenerative changes are found in the kidneys, liver, stomach and heart, and a considerable amount of arsenic may be found in the liver and less in the kidney.

Atrophy and degeneration is sometimes found in the spinal cord and especially in the cells in the anterior horn of the grey matter. Neuritis with degeneration of the myelin may be found in the peripheral nerves, and the axis cylinders may also be involved.

In medico-legal cases, where the post-mortem has to be done after exhumation of the body, it is always advisable to take some of the soil lying, not in contact with, but in the vicinity of, the body, and to examine this for the presence of arsenic, lest the arsenic may have diffused into the body from without. It is extremely unlikely that much arsenic will get into the organs in this way, but experimentally this diffusion has been found to be possible, and therefore it is important to have evidence on this point in any given case.

Antimony (Tartar emetic). This, like arsenic, acts as a special irritant of the gastro-intestinal tract. The œsophagus, the stomach and the duodenum suffer most in the *acute* cases. The mucous membrane of these regions, as well as that of the pharynx, is congested, inflamed and œdematous, and ulcerated patches which may expose the muscular coats may be developed. There are usually submucous hæmorrhages and the stomach may contain tenacious, dark or blood-stained mucus. The changes may be most marked at the cardiac end, but usually are found throughout the stomach. In some of the recorded cases no visible changes were found post-mortem.

Chronic poisoning. There may be very little evidence of any special pathological change, though in some cases ulcers may be found in the stomach, in the cæcum or in the colon. The kidneys and liver may shew fatty or other degenerative changes.

Chloride of antimony produces post-mortem appearances like those of a corrosive, such as hydrochloric acid.

Mercury, copper and zinc. In acute cases of poisoning with these substances, the main pathological appearance is an intense gastro-enteritis. In the mouth, the pharynx and the œsophagus, the epithelium becomes swollen, greyish in colour and sodden in appearance. More marked changes of an inflammatory nature, with extravasation of blood and softening and even ulceration of the mucous membrane, are found in the stomach and in the intestines. Wide spread superficial necrosis with ulceration and hæmorrhages in the large intestine is a characteristic feature in acute mercurial poisoning. Perforation of the stomach or of the intestine is not common but may occur, but irregular contractions of the muscular wall of the bowel are frequent.

In cases of *copper poisoning* the wall of the stomach is usually of a bluish (with the sulphate) or greenish (with the acetate) colour, and the superficial epithelium is dark brown ; with *mercury* the mucous membrane is greyish-white unless in cases where there has been previous congestion and then the colour may be bluish-grey ; with *zinc* there are no special colour changes.

Again in cases of *zinc poisoning* the pathological appearances vary with the salt that is used. *Zinc sulphate* acts like an irritant poison and the changes are those of a very acute gastro-enteritis, whereas with *zinc chloride* the corrosive action is more pronounced and the necrosis is more intense than the inflammatory reaction—the mucous membrane becomes white, opaque and readily detached, and the wall of the stomach hard and leathery.

Changes in the other organs. The liver shows fatty and other degenerative changes. In the kidneys, in addition to the fatty changes, there is usually a marked necrosis in the secreting cells, especially in case of mercurial poisoning. Calcareous deposit in these degenerated cells is a characteristic feature of poisoning with mercurial salts. In one case, in which I did the post-mortem examination, this was very marked, though the poisoning arose from *intrauterine douching* with perchloride of mercury.

Chronic poisoning. This is not common with these substances and, where it does occur, the main pathological changes are inflammatory reactions and even ulceration in the lower part of the colon and in the rectum. In some cases the cæcum is also involved. Workers with mercury may develop fine tremor of the muscles and sensory symptoms associated with disease of the nervous system, but no definite post-mortem evidence of gross changes has been brought forward.

Lead. Poisoning with *lead* usually occurs in a chronic form, and there are no pathological changes which are definitely diagnostic of the condition. The gums may become spongy, swollen and hæmorrhagic and there may be a " blue line " at the junction of the gums and the teeth, especially in the lower jaw. Chronic gastric catarrh and chronic enteritis with associated pigmentation of the mucous membrane may be present. Degenerative changes may be found in the brain and in the spinal cord, and considerable overgrowth of fibrous tissue is usually present in the kidneys in very chronic cases. The granular contracted kidney, which is sometimes associated with chronic lead poisoning, may be due to the action of the lead on the kidney itself, or to arterio-sclerotic changes. There is, however, no very definite evidence that lead can of itself produce this arterial degeneration. Lead salts are excreted by both the bowel and the kidneys.

In *acute poisoning* gastro-enteritis of varying degrees of intensity is the main post-mortem manifestation.

Silver. Acute silver poisoning is extremely uncommon—the silver salt acts as an irritant in the stomach and the intestine. The exposed parts of the lips and mouth may shew dark staining due to the action of light on the salt employed.

In *chronic* cases the main change is a darkening of the exposed parts of the body due to the deposit of metallic silver in the superficial layers of the skin and mucous membranes. This deposit is also seen in the sweat glands and in the kidneys after exposure to light.

Phosphorus. In *acute* cases there may be evidence of slight acute congestion of the whole intestinal tract or there may be more extensive changes producing swelling and extensive fatty degeneration of the mucous membrane. Ecchymosis and superficial erosions may be present. The stomach may contain dark fluid which has a garlic odour, especially if heated. Extensive fatty changes occur in the liver, giving it a bright yellow colour and causing considerable enlargement. Similar fatty changes, though usually not so pronounced, are found in the kidneys, in the heart, in the voluntary muscles and in the endothelium of the vessels. Microscopical examination should be made of the various organs so that the situation in which the fat occurs may be determined. Diffuse scattered hæmorrhages in the heart and in the serous membranes are common and these are probably associated with the fatty changes in the endothelium of the vessels. Jaundice is common and is caused by obstruction of the small bile capillaries by swollen and degenerated cells and by inspissated mucus. The condition should be carefully differentiated from acute yellow atrophy, where the liver is reduced in size, firm and of a dark yellow colour.

Chronic phosphorus poisoning. The characteristic change is necrosis of the bones of the upper and lower jaw—especially of the latter.

Chloroform. *Acute* poisoning by drinking liquid chloroform is so rare that it need only be mentioned. The lesions produced will be swelling and superficial necrosis of the mucous membrane of the pharynx, œsophagus and stomach.

Deaths from inhalation of chloroform vapour usually shew no characteristic post-mortem appearances. In cases of *delayed chloroform poisoning*, there is extensive fatty degeneration, resembling that seen in phosphorus poisoning. The liver is enlarged, of a canary yellow colour and intensely fatty. The heart and the kidneys shew similar changes though in a lessened degree. The mucous and serous membranes may shew hæmorrhages. The fatty changes may be less marked in one case than in another, but in the liver are always very evident.

In cases of *septic poisoning* the fatty changes may also be very pronounced, and in suspected cases of delayed chloroform poisoning it is extremely important to examine for any septic focus and to make a bacteriological examination of that area and also of the blood from the heart. As I have pointed out elsewhere, an examination of the bone marrow should also be made. There *may* be no leucoblastic reaction in chloroform cases, but the reaction is always present in septic cases, if the bone marrow was previously healthy.

Potassium nitrate (saltpetre) gives rise to acute gastritis, and *potassium chlorate* causes the mucous membrane of the stomach to be swollen, softened and separated. The blood is inspissated and dark brown in colour, giving the spectroscopic reactions of methæmoglobin. The kidneys are chocolate coloured, and on microscopical examination shew a reddish-brown deposit of altered blood in the cloudy epithelium of the secreting tubules.

Hydrocyanic acid and *cyanide of potassium*. The mucous membrane of the stomach may be bright red and congested, and petechial hæmorrhages may be present, but there are no post-mortem appearances which are characteristic. The odour of the hydrocyanic acid may sometimes be detected.

Alcohol. In *acute* poisoning there is congestion of the mucous membrane of the stomach with increased secretion of mucus ; in *chronic* cases there is evidence of chronic gastric catarrh, but no definite diagnosis of alcoholic poisoning can be given on post-mortem evidence alone. There may be cirrhosis of the liver ; fatty and other degenerative changes in the liver, in the heart and in the kidneys ; atheroma in the vessels ; chronic degenerative and hyperplastic changes in the kidney and degenerative changes in the pia mater and in the brain ; but it is not uncommon to find comparatively little pathological change in cases of chronic alcoholism.

Chloral hydrate, iodoform and ether poisoning sometimes occur, but the pathological appearances in these cases are not in any way characteristic. There may be congestion of the mucous membranes of the œsophagus and stomach, and fatty degeneration may occur in the liver and in the kidneys, but these changes are not constant and, besides, they are frequently associated with and caused by other organic and inorganic poisons.

Other substances which may act as irritant poisons. Chromic acid, bromine and iodine may produce very little post-mortem changes, but some signs of inflammation such as swelling and separation of the superficial epithelium may be found. The tissues which have been in contact with the poison may be stained yellow with chromic acid or with iodine, and brown with bromine. The odour of the bromine or of the iodine may be detected in some cases.

POISONING WITH GASES.

Carbonic acid gas (carbon dioxide). Death takes place from asphyxia. The face is livid and swollen, the lungs *may* shew congestion and hæmorrhages, the right heart is distended, and there may be small superficial hæmorrhages in the meninges and in the brain itself. Similar appearances may be found in cases of poisoning with *carbon bisulphide, sulphuretted hydrogen, sewer gas,* though in all of these, the changes in the lungs are usually more marked—evidence of congestion, œdema, catarrhal changes and even pneumonia being sometimes found. In poisoning with *sulphuretted hydrogen* putrefactive changes quickly follow death and the blood is dark in colour and on spectroscopic examination shews a narrow line towards the red end of the spectrum, between C and D, resembling that of hæmoglobin, but which does not disappear on the addition of a reducing agent, as the methæmoglobin band does when similarly treated.

From what has been said it will be seen that no specially characteristic pathological changes, apart from those due to death from asphyxia, are likely to be noticed at the post-mortem examination in deaths due to this group of poisons.

Carbon monoxide. In acute poisoning with carbon monoxide the face, the neck, the chest and the thighs are of a rosy-red tint, and the blood throughout the body is similar in appearance, and it has a diminished coagulation index. The lungs are usually congested and œdematous, and shew the same rosy-red colour, which is also seen in the muscles. The presence of carbon monoxide in the blood can be detected by spectroscopic examination. If a drop of sulphide of ammonium be added to diluted normal blood, the two oxyhæmoglobin bands between *D* and *E* disappear, and one band—that characteristic of reduced hæmoglobin—is seen. Glaister states that if carbon monoxide blood is treated in a similar manner, no alteration takes place. Again, if a drop of normal blood is diluted with saline until the mixture appears of a yellow colour, and then an equal amount of saline is added to a drop of carbon monoxide blood, the yellow colour does not appear—the carbon monoxide blood still retains its rosy-red colour.

In cases of poisoning by *water gas, illuminating gas*, and the gases produced by explosions of *gunpowder* and *nitro-glycerine*, and possibly other explosives, the deaths are generally due to the carbon monoxide or carbon dioxide which is present in the gas.

Arseniuretted hydrogen gas. Dixon-Mann states that chemical analysis will reveal the presence of arsenic in the tissues. The mucous membrane of the stomach and small intestine is deeply congested and petechial hæmorrhages are common. The lungs are œdematous and the liver and kidneys shew cloudy swelling and fatty degeneration. The viscera are generally tinged bluish-black and jaundice is present.

CARBON COMPOUNDS.

Benzene. There may be a slight smell of benzene on opening the body, inflammation of the œsophageal and gastric mucous membrane with erosions may be present, and the lungs may shew congestion and purulent bronchitis. On the other hand no definite pathological changes may be found.

Nitro-benzene. Similar post-mortem appearances may be found as are seen in cases of poisoning with benzene, and death is usually due to asphyxia. The blood may be dark and chocolate coloured, and ecchymoses have been found in the mucous membranes.

Poisonings by *anilin, pyridine, antifebrin, antipyrin, phenacetin, naphthalene, resorcin*, etc. so rarely end fatally that very little knowledge is possessed as to the pathological changes which they produce.

Carbolic acid. Stains produced by the poison may be present about the mouth. The mucous membrane of the mouth, pharynx and œsophagus may be softened and of a dull-grey colour, and the mucous membrane of the stomach may shew a similar appearance, or it may be corrugated, hardened and of a brown colour. Small hæmorrhagic foci are present and blood-stained mucus is found in the stomach, but actual erosion is uncommon. The duodenum may present a similar appearance.

Creosote. The post-mortem changes are similar to those seen in carbolic acid poisoning.

ALKALOIDS AND VEGETABLE POISONS.

Strychnine. Sometimes post-mortem rigidity is prolonged, but this is not invariable. Death usually results from asphyxia and there are no characteristic post-mortem changes.

Opium and morphine. There are no characteristic post-mortem changes. The odour may be perceptible. In some cases, but by no means in all, there is congestion of the gastric mucous membrane and also of the brain, and there may be œdema into the subarachnoid space and the ventricles. Death is usually from asphyxia, and the blood is therefore usually dark and fluid.

Atropine and belladonna. If the belladonna berries have been eaten, there may be congestion of the mucous membrane of the stomach, and search should be made in the stomach and in the intestines for the seeds. No other post-mortem changes are seen, and in many cases of poisoning with the drugs there are no characteristic changes. Death is from asphyxia.

Cocaine. The principal changes are hyperæmia of the membranes of the brain and cord, and of the viscera generally. Death is from asphyxia.

Of the *other vegetable poisons* nothing need be said. The post-mortem appearances are not characteristic, and chemical examination alone is of value in determining their presence in the alimentary canal or in the tissues.

Poisonous fungi. There may be considerable inflammation of the gastro-intestinal mucous membrane with hæmorrhagic spots and erosions. Petechial hæmorrhages occur in the pleura and pericardium. The heart and the other organs are often engorged with dark coloured blood, and fatty degeneration is seen in the liver, heart and kidneys.

ANIMAL POISONS.

Cantharides. The mucous membrane of the digestive tract may be swollen and inflamed, and erosions and ulcers may be present. This condition will be most marked in the upper part of the tract but may extend as far as the rectum. If the powdered insect has been swallowed careful examination of the mucous membrane with a lens should be made in order to detect any bright glistening portions of the fly. The kidneys usually are swollen and shew extensive necrosis in the epithelial cells of the tubules, and the inner coats of the bladder and urethra may be congested.

CHAPTER XII

BACTERIOLOGICAL EXAMINATION

I. METHODS FOR THE BACTERIOLOGICAL EXAMINATION OF LABORATORY ANIMALS

Many bacteriologists recommend that the animal should be dipped in or washed with some antiseptic solution, such as corrosive sublimate or lysol, before the post-mortem is begun. This is largely to prevent hair or wool being disseminated through the laboratory, but it also serves to destroy fleas or other external parasites which might convey infection—*e.g.* plague—to the operator. If the post-mortem is done with care this procedure is quite satisfactory, but the worker must always remember that if the antiseptic reaches the area which he wishes to examine bacteriologically his results may be entirely negative, merely because he has introduced some of the antiseptic into his culture tubes.

Personally I prefer to moisten the hair or wool very thoroughly with sterilised water or, if there is any probable risk of infection by external parasites, the animal may be put into a dish of petrol for five minutes. The general method of examination is similar to that carried out in the human subject and the area which requires examination is generally well defined—thus the blood or the spleen in anthrax, the lymphatic glands in tuberculosis where the injection has been into the subcutaneous tissues, etc.

For this examination I always use instruments which are sterilised in the flame immediately before use. They are usually blunt and not so easy to work with, but their sterility is more certain and this is the point of primary importance in this work. The animal should always be pinned out before commencing the examination—that part to which special attention is directed being placed most conveniently for the operator. The skin is reflected from the area to be examined, and then the superficial tissues over a fairly wide area are thoroughly seared with a cautery. The thorax or the abdomen is now opened by an incision which gives free access to the part which requires special examination.

The thorax. Any fluid in the pleural cavities is withdrawn into a sterile pipette and inoculated at once into a tube of suitable media. The pericardium is opened with sterile scissors and the surface of the heart over a small area is seared. Through the sterilised area a sterile pipette is introduced into one of the cavities and a quantity of blood is sucked up. This is then inoculated into a culture tube. The lungs and the heart may now be removed, opened up and examined—sterile instruments being used—and any diseased area which is found can be examined bacteriologically if the operator thinks this advisable.

The abdomen. Procedure similar to that adopted for the thorax is employed—any fluid which is present is withdrawn into a suitable sterile pipette and inoculated into tubes of suitable media. If bacteriological examinations of the liver, spleen, kidneys, etc. are required, these organs are first removed and placed in a sterile dish, and the surface, or a part of it, thoroughly seared so as to destroy any bacteria which have lodged there. The organ is then cut into with a sterile knife or torn across, and small pieces taken from various parts are first crushed carefully and inoculated in suitable media. Films and sections should also be made in special cases, *e.g.* tuberculosis, plague, etc.

Abscess cavities, suppurative foci, etc., whether present in the walls or in the internal organs, should be examined both by films and by culture.

Enlarged glands. Examination of these may be of primary importance, *e.g.* in cases of tuberculosis, plague, and glanders. The gland should be excised with sterile precautions and placed in a sterile dish. It should then be cut carefully in various directions with a sterile knife, and the various portions rubbed on to suitable solid media or placed in fluid media. The more detailed examination in cases such as have been referred to here—tuberculosis, plague and glanders—will be found in later chapters.

Cobbett and Graham Smith (*Journal of Hygiene*, vol. x No. 1) give very careful instructions for making cultures from the organs of birds. Though some of the precautions they take may not be necessary in many cases, their instructions are so extremely good that, even at the risk of repeating many points I have already made, I propose quoting their statements in full.

" 1. *Precautions against aerial contamination.*

Previous to beginning an experiment the room was carefully prepared. All dust was removed from the window ledges and elsewhere, and the floor and bench were flooded with a mixture of glycerine and lysol to lay the dust. All the windows and ventilation shafts were closed during the actual operation of making the cultures. As a further precaution against aerial contamination the tissues were crushed inside a glass frame. Two sheets of plate glass, 21 × 8 inches, formed the top and bottom respectively, the former being supported on blocks of wood, which formed the sides. The back was also formed of a sheet of plate glass, and the front was closed by a curtain of linen, which was soaked in lysol and could be partially turned back when required. The joints of the frame were made draught proof by means of rubber tubing. On the floor of the frame another sheet of plate glass, which extended the whole length, but was three inches narrower than the bottom, was placed to form a ledge near the centre of the floor, upon which the plates used for crushing the tissues could be conveniently manipulated, and yet be covered by the roof. The height of the frame from the top to this ledge was three and a half inches.

Before using, the frame was washed out with a mixture of glycerine and lysol. In order to estimate the risk of aerial contamination agar plates were exposed on the bench and inside the frame during the whole period of time the cultures were being made.

2. *The preparation of the bird.*

The birds, if living, were killed by decapitation, weighed and immediately plucked in an adjoining room. As far as possible all the larger feathers, except those of the wings, were removed, and the cloaca, if gaping, was plugged with a pledget of cotton wool. The smaller feathers appeared to us to be a particularly dangerous source of contamination, since some might be soiled with faecal matter. Owing to their extreme lightness some of these unless carefully destroyed might float in the air and alight on the tissues during the manipulations. The smallest feathers are seen only with difficulty, and might easily contaminate pieces of tissue as they were being removed from the body. In order to obviate all chance of contamination from feathers the body of the bird after plucking was held in the flame until all the minute feathers had been completely destroyed.

3. *The method of obtaining portions of the organs.*

A plumber's soldering-iron, heated to redness, was freely used to burn the skin through which the incisions for removing

pieces of tissue were to be made.   The necessary incisions were
then made without delay with instruments sterilised by boiling
for at least half-an-hour.   A fresh pair of scissors and forceps
were used for removing the piece of tissue actually used for
cultivation.   Cultivations were made from each organ in turn,
observing the precautions which have just been described in
each case. *Lungs.*—The lungs were approached from the back.
After the skin had been thoroughly seared with the iron the
muscles under the scapula were transfixed with a knife and the
scapula freed by carrying the knife out to its apex ; the bone
was then turned up and broken.   Next two or more ribs were
cut through in two places, about half an inch apart, with scissors,
and a piece of the lung approximately equal in bulk to a cube
one-quarter of an inch in all dimensions was cut out, and quickly
transferred to the ground glass plates for disintegration.
Kidneys.—As the kidneys were approached from the back they
were taken immediately after the lungs.   A piece of the thin
iliac bone, where it bulges outwards, was removed, care being
taken not to force the intestines upwards during the process
by pressure on the body.   The satisfactory removal of portions
of the kidneys was often a difficult matter, partly owing to the
limited size of the opening which could be conveniently made
in the bone, and partly owing to the nerve trunks which traverse
the organs and render the extraction of portions difficult.   In
a few cases the intestine was wounded, but when this accident
was perceived at once the attempt to obtain any further cultures
from this bird was abandoned. *Liver, Pancreas and Spleen.*—
These organs were approached from the front by turning the
sternum back after cauterising the whole ventral surface, and
especially the lines of the incision.   Culture tubes were always
sown from the liver, but the pancreas was only examined cul-
turally on a few occasions, and cultures from the spleen were
not made when the organ was required for histological purposes.
In the grouse the spleen is extremely small, so that even when
cultures were made the amount of material employed was
considerably less than in the case of other organs. *Blood and
Bile.*—Samples of blood were obtained by plunging sterile
pipettes through the heart wall after cauterisation.   Bile was

also obtained in glass pipettes from the gall bladder, but the surface of the latter organ was not cauterised.

4. *The method of crushing the tissues.*

From each organ a piece, at least a quarter of an inch square, was removed by the methods just described, and placed on the surface of a ground glass plate. The plates used were 3 to 4 inches in diameter and were ground on one side ; these were sterilised by boiling and dried separately in the flame. As soon as they were dry the plates were placed in pairs, with their ground surfaces in contact on the glass ledge which has been described in the glass frame ; in this situation they cooled rapidly. When a portion of an organ was ready to be ground up the upper plate of a pair was taken up and held in the fingers in such a way that about one-half or one-quarter of it over-lapped an equal area of the lower plate. The piece of tissue was then placed between the overlapping areas and crushed. It was not found necessary to use powdered glass or other material to assist disintegration, because the organs of the bird, protected as they are from violence by the comparatively rigid skeleton, are much softer than those of mammals, and are easily reduced to the condition of an emulsion.

5. *The method of making cultures.*

Before starting an experiment a series of sloped agar tubes were labelled, two or three for each organ, and arranged on the bench in the order in which the organs were to be dealt with. As soon as a portion of an organ had been reduced to a pulp a considerable quantity of the pulp was taken up on a sterile platinum wire, bent into a series of loops so as to form a spatula, and spread over the surface of one of the agar tubes. The whole of the material crushed was left on the two tubes. In this way any living organisms that might be present had an opportunity of producing colonies on the surface of the medium. In the case of 9 birds (Nos. 20—28) anaerobic cultures in Buchner tubes were also made from all the organs, but as they did not yield anything more than the ordinary cultures, such cultures were not made in the later experiments.

6. *The examination of cultures.*

The cultures were incubated at 37° C. and examined daily on the first few days, and subsequently at various intervals up to a fortnight. Colonies of *B. coli* or *streptococci* seldom appeared after 24—48 hours' cultivation, except when they grew out of one of the larger masses of tissue on the surface of the tube. The principal result of allowing the cultures to incubate for longer periods was to reveal the presence of moulds and streptothrices, and occasional spore-bearing bacilli and cocci in cultures from the lungs.

The examination of the agar plates, exposed on the bench and within the glass frame during the progress of the experiments, shewed that in spite of the long exposure very few colonies grew on them. *B. coli* was never found and moulds and streptothrices were uncommon. The commonest organisms were *S. lutea* and cocci."

2. HISTOLOGICAL AND BACTERIOLOGICAL EXAMINATION IN MAN.

In describing the general post-mortem methods, it was pointed out that portions of any fluid found in the pleural or pericardial cavities, in the peritoneal sac, in the cavities of the joints, in the cavities of the brain and spinal cord or elsewhere, and of any inflammatory exudate should be collected in sterile tubes and left for subsequent histological and bacteriological examination. If the fluid is small in amount or if the exudate is scanty, inoculations on various media may be made at once. At the conclusion of the post-mortem examination, inoculations from any fluid or exudate which has been collected should be made in nutrient broth or on nutrient agar, or on that media which is known to be most suitable for the growth of the organism whose presence is suspected. The details of the methods for doing these bacteriological tests, and the special media which in any individual case is most useful, cannot be fully described in this manual, though reference will be made to some of the more important methods and media in the chapters dealing with special diseases and in the appendix. For full details, however, reference should be made to books dealing more specifically with bacteriology.

In certain cases, *e.g.* suspected tuberculosis, plague, pneumococcal infections, etc., it may be advisable or indeed essential that some of the fluid or exudate should be inoculated into guinea-pigs, mice, rabbits, etc.

For *histological* examination of the fluids and other exudates films should be made either before or after centrifugalisation, and these stained with some appropriate stain—*e.g.* hæmatein and eosin for cells, Leishman's stain, thionin blue, methylene blue, carbol-fuchsin, etc. for bacteria and protozoa.

Examination of the individual organs and tissues. The greatest care must be taken to avoid extraneous contamination whether from the air, the skin or elsewhere. It will be impossible to carry out all the details which are recorded under the heading " Methods for the bacteriological examination of laboratory animals " on p. 138, but the more essential of these precautions should on no account be omitted.

The heart. Bacteriological examination will mainly be concerned with the blood, vegetations on the valves and abscesses or other septic condition in the muscle. For the examination of the blood the surface of the right ventricle about its centre should be seared with a hot knife, or preferably a small soldering iron, over an area about ½ to 1 inch square. A sterilised pipette with a fine bore should be plunged through the muscle in the centre of the seared area, into the cavity of the right ventricle. (The open end of the pipette should be plugged loosely with cotton wool, before it is sterilised.) By slight suction blood or serum can be drawn up into the pipette and immediately inoculated into a suitable media—either nutrient broth or nutrient agar being most commonly used.

Vegetations on the valves. These are examined after the heart is removed, and they should be looked for preliminary to opening the cavities and before any water test for competency has been tried. Vegetations on the mitral valves can generally be detected by an examination of the mitral orifice through the left auricle, and on the aortic valves they may be seen directly, if the coronary arteries are slit up in the method which I have described. Small portions of the vegetations should be removed with a pair of dissecting forceps whose points have been sterilised in the flame, rather than with a platinum needle, which is often too delicate for firm vegetations —and the portion inoculated in nutrient broth, in milk or other suitable media. The principal organisms to be considered are streptococci and pneumococci, though others may be found. If the orifices have been opened up before the vegetations are discovered, small portions should be taken from the less exposed areas, or if possible from the deeper parts after the surface has been seared with a fine wire or with the narrow end of the blade of the forceps.

Abscess or other septic condition in the muscle. The surface of the affected area is seared, an incision made into it with a sterile knife, and a scraping taken either with the knife or with a platinum loop, and this material inoculated on to suitable media.

The lungs. If examination of the contents of the bronchi is deemed necessary, some of the secretion is taken from the deeper and less exposed parts with a platinum loop, and films made, and the secretion is inoculated on to suitable culture media. For general use nutrient agar is most valuable, but blood agar may be necessary in cases of influenza or pneumococcal infection, and blood serum in diphtheritic conditions.

If any area in the substance of the lung requires special examination, the superficial part is thoroughly seared with a soldering iron and a piece of tissue cut out with a sterile knife or a sterile pair of scissors. The size of this piece of tissue will vary with the condition found. It may be small where a suppurative foci is seen or it may be at least half-an-inch square. The piece of tissue is either inoculated directly into fluid media or put into a sterile Petri dish and thoroughly crushed before being smeared over the surface of solid media.

Films should be made at the same time and either dried or fixed with some chemical fixative such as formalin, alcohol, etc., and then stained with the most appropriate solution. For the histological structure of cells hæmatein and eosin or some modification of this double staining is the most valuable, whilst for bacteria any of the aniline stains are useful.

Bacteriological examination of any other of the thoracic or cervical tissues is performed in a similar manner. In all these manipulations I prefer to use instruments which have been sterilised in the naked flame immediately before use.

Before completing the examination, small portions of all the organs and the tissues should be cut off and placed in some fixing solution for careful microscopical investigation. The area from which these portions are to be cut must of course be determined by the site of the pathological change, and by the experience of the pathologist as to the position in which he is most likely to find any morbid conditions. It is quite impossible to give definite directions in the majority of cases.

The liver, the spleen, the kidneys, and the pancreas. Abscesses in any of these organs are carefully looked for ; if they are large the surface is seared with the soldering iron and the pus withdrawn into a sterile pipette which has been plunged through the wall in the centre of the seared area, or an incision may be made over the seared area and a sterile swab introduced ; if the abscess is small its superficial wall and the adjacent tissue is seared, the abscess is cut into with a sterile knife and inoculations are made on suitable media with a looped platinum needle.

Where the pathological area is solid or where there is no obvious area of disease, portions of the organ about one-quarter to half-an-inch square should be cut out either from the obviously diseased part or from several separate areas. In order to do this satisfactorily I recommend that the surface of the organ should be thoroughly seared with the soldering iron over one or more areas. These are then cut into with a sterile knife and the organ so folded that it will tear slightly ; a portion about a quarter of an inch square is then cut out from this freshly-exposed surface, crushed in a sterile Petri dish and inoculated on the surface of solid media or placed whole into a tube of fluid media. Where there are no obvious pathological changes, pieces of tissue from several different areas should be examined, otherwise the organisms may be entirely missed.

Suprarenals, mesenteric and other lymphatic glands, thryoid, thymus, etc. These organs are very carefully seared, either over the whole surface, if the gland is small, or over a sufficiently large area to enable a portion of about one-eighth to a quarter of an inch in diameter to be cut out with sterile scissors. This piece of tissue, which must not include any external surface which has not been well burned with the soldering iron, and the whole of any small gland are put into a sterile Petri dish and carefully chopped up and then crushed before inoculation on to the surface of a tube of suitable media. The whole of the gland or the piece of tissue may be cut into in several places and inoculated directly into a tube of fluid media.

Small blocks of tissue about one-quarter of an inch in diameter are cut from all these solid organs and put into some fixative solution for later examination for histological structure. The portion from which the block shall be cut must, of course, be determined by the character of the morbid condition present, and by the general pathological knowledge of the operator.

The mouth, the pharynx, the larynx and the œsophagus. Bacteriological examination of these regions is usually undertaken because of the presence of some acute or chronic inflammatory, necrotic or suppurative condition, or of some fibrinous or other deposit on the surface—*e.g.* the membrane in diphtheria or in septic pharyngitis, or the fungus in cases of stomatitis. Scrapings may be made from the membranes, from the suppurative or ulcerated lesions, or from any other pathological area, by means of a platinum needle, and inoculated directly on to suitable culture media, but it is generally more convenient to rub over the surface or push into the abscess cavity a sterile cotton-wool swab, which is then put into a sterile tube for later examination both by cultural methods and by means of films on glass slides.

It may be desirable in certain cases to examine ulcerated

areas or swollen patches or even caseous or necrotic tonsils or other glands for the presence of *B. tuberculosis* or for the *spirochæta pallida*. This may be done by section-method or by scrapings which are fixed and stained with appropriate stains (see Appendix). Inoculation of any secretion or of any caseous material may be necessary, but the knowledge and judgement of the pathologist must be the guide in any given case. No specially useful purpose will be served by attempting to cultivate directly either *B. tuberculosis* or *spirochæta pallida*.

Finally portions of tissue which shew any pathological changes should be put aside in some fixative solution for subsequent histological examination.

Stomach and intestines. In certain cases it may be necessary to sear the surface, to make an incision and cut out or scrape out some tissue from the unexposed parts and inoculate this in suitable media—*e.g.* in cases of phlegmonous gastritis. More commonly, however, scrapings are taken directly from the damaged area, *e.g.* the ulcerated swollen areas in typhoid fever, dysentery, ulcerative colitis, etc., and inoculated on plates of suitable media. Later, detailed examination is carried out, and the colonies of different organisms separated and carefully examined. This is sometimes a matter of great difficulty, and the process is generally tedious and requires to be done by a skilled bacteriologist.

Areas of suspected tuberculosis or syphilis are examined by scrapings, which are spread on glass slides and examined by the routine staining methods, and in some cases histological examination by sections, and even inoculation into animals may be necessary.

In special cases, *e.g.* typhoid fever, it is often important to examine bacteriologically certain regions such as the gall bladder and the spleen, but such cases will be dealt with in later chapters, for at present only those fundamental details which are necessary for a successful bacteriological examination are being discussed.

Gall bladder and urinary bladder. The outer surface should be seared, the cavity opened through the sterilised area and the fluid withdrawn into a sterile pipette and inoculated

in suitable fluid media or plated out on solid media. The
cavity should then be opened more widely and scrapings taken
from the mucous membrane, from ulcerated or inflamed areas,
from abscesses, etc., and inoculated in agar, litmus dextrose or
other appropriate media.

Genital organs. The examination of these is carried out
exactly in the manner described for solid organs such as glands,
liver, etc., it being always remembered that the flora of the
vagina and sometimes of the uterus is profuse and that many
of the organisms have no pathological significance.

Arteries and veins. The most important condition which
requires bacteriological examination is thrombosis. The wall
of the vessel may be seared, then opened, and a portion of the
thrombus inoculated on to solid or fluid media. Examination
of the deeper layers of the intima of arteries has been carried
out in connection with degenerative changes ; the inner surface
is seared and a thin-bladed knife (such as a cataract knife)
is carefully introduced under the superficial layers of the intima,
and scrapings made with this and these inoculated in broth
or on agar or gelatine.

The brain and the spinal cord. Two classes of cases call
for special bacteriological examination :

(*a*) Those caused by bacteria which, by their action, produce
serous or purulent exudate, etc. in and under the membranes
or in the substance of the brain.

(*b*) Those which are infective, but for which no definite
causal organism has been discovered.

For the former type of cases it is usually sufficient to inoculate tubes directly from the exudate or from softened or degenerated areas or to collect some of the exudate, etc. in sterile
tubes for subsequent examination. In many cases, and particularly in cerebro-spinal meningitis it is essential to inoculate
the tubes at the examination, or as early as possible afterwards.

In certain cases, *e.g.* in tuberculous meningitis, pneumococcal infections, etc., it may be desirable to inoculate the
exudate directly into guinea-pigs, rabbits or mice, or this may
be required at a later period of the examination in order to
arrive at a correct diagnosis of the organism which was present.

For the latter type of case, *e.g.* hydrophobia and infantile paralysis, extract or filtered extract of the brain or of the spinal cord may be injected directly into animals. The methods will be described in Chapter XIV.

Portions of the brain and the spinal cord which shew, or are likely to shew, pathological changes should be removed and put in fixative solution for subsequent histological examination.

Bones and joints. Bone conditions, other than suppuration and caries or necrosis, rarely call for bacteriological examination, but where necessary portions of the softened tissue or purulent exudate are scraped away and tubes of media either inoculated directly from the material or kept in a sterile tube for subsequent examination at the laboratory.

Joints are opened carefully—the skin is first reflected from the affected joint, the subcutaneous tissues thoroughly seared and an incision made into the joint with a sterile knife. If fluid is present, this may be collected in a sterile tube or on a sterile swab, but pieces of the synovial membrane should also be removed at a number of different areas in the joint cavity. Tubes may be inoculated at the examination or at a later period. Fluid media should be employed for culture from the portions of the synovial membrane.

In my experience the synovial membrane is usually found to be sterile except in cases of septicæmia or where putrefactive changes have taken place in the body. Where I have succeeded in isolating pathogenetic organisms, which were not present in the circulating blood, it has been found necessary to examine several pieces of the membrane from different areas in the larger joints, and from the smaller joints to cut off with bone forceps the ends of the bones and introduce these, with the synovial membrane, into large tubes. In inflammatory conditions, areas of congestion may be seen in the synovial membrane, and such areas are, of course, cut out for bacteriological examination. Fringes from overgrown synovial membranes and nodules of bony overgrowth should also be cut away and put into tubes of fluid media.

Histological examination may be necessary in some cases,

and portions of bone, etc. should be put in some fixative solution (see Appendix).

The nasal cavities, the external and middle ear, etc. These and other cavities present no special difficulties in examination, but it is essential that they should be thoroughly opened up lest some small collection of pus or other infective material be overlooked. The secretion or other pathological material should be collected on a sterile swab and this reserved for subsequent inoculation, etc.

Where masses of granulation tissue or tumours occur, portions of these should be removed for histological examination in order to determine not only their morbid histological structure but the presence of parasites, *e.g. spirochæta, rhinosporidium,* etc.

CHAPTER XIII

EXAMINATION OF SPECIAL CASES

The general procedure in any given case will be that already described, but modifications will be necessary, special situations may call for particular examination and special procedure, particularly in regard to bacteriological examination, may be advisable in individual cases. It must however be clearly understood that the examination of special areas cannot be substituted for an exhaustive examination in every case where that is possible. It frequently happens, however, that permission for a limited examination only is given, or that the operator has not sufficient time for a complete examination and that he must content himself with observations on the essential lesions in the case at the post-mortem table, so that afterwards he may be able more fully to work out the case in the laboratory. For this purpose it seems necessary to give some detailed information as to the special lesions which require examination in special cases, and the methods to be employed, not only at the time of the examination, but subsequently in the laboratory. Necessarily, in such a book as the present, information as to

laboratory procedure must be confined to simple routine
methods, and for the more elaborate processes reference must
be made to text-books on bacteriology or on bacteriological
and pathological technique.

In all cases where sepsis is probable, examination of the
blood in the heart should be made by cultural methods. After
opening the pericardium, the surface of the right ventricle
over a area about one inch square is seared and a sterile pipette,
plugged with cotton-wool at the outer end, is plunged through
the wall and a few cubic centimetres of blood drawn into it.
This blood is then introduced into tubes of broth, or other
suitable media.

Diphtheria, Scarlet Fever, Measles.

In these diseases the post-mortem examination is conducted
in the ordinary way, but the lungs are specially examined for
areas of broncho-pneumonia and associated collapse ; and
the naso-pharynx, larynx and bronchi are searched for any
evidence of membrane. The greyish membrane which is most
characteristic in diphtheria may be present in both scarlet
fever and measles. The middle ear should also be examined
for muco-purulent or purulent secretion. The lymphatic
glands, especially those at the angle of the jaw are cut into
and any evidence of inflammation or suppuration noted.

In diphtheria, the heart should always be examined for
evidence of fatty degeneration, and myocarditis may sometimes
be present ; in scarlet fever careful examination of the heart
should be made for evidence of pericarditis and endocarditis.
The kidneys may shew degenerative changes in the secreting
cells or even extensive changes in the glomeruli, and in the
interstitial tissue, and it is always very important in these
diseases to systematically examine, by microscopical methods,
the kidneys. In measles, especially, any evidence of tuberculosis should be sought for, and this may be exhibited in the
bronchial glands alone or in the lungs as a tuberculous broncho-
pneumonia, or as a generalised miliary tuberculosis. The
tonsils and the lymphatic glands at the angles of the jaw should

be examined microscopically for signs of tuberculosis. The other organs and tissues do not usually shew any specially characteristic lesions, but if symptoms indicating involvement of the nervous system have been present, the brain and the spinal cord should be carefully examined.

Bacteriological examination of any membrane that may be present, of any purulent or semi-purulent exudate, of inflamed glands and of broncho-pneumonic patches in the lungs, should be undertaken.

From any membrane that is present cultures should be made on solidified blood serum, on nasgar and on ordinary agar, and the growths examined by film preparations in from 12 to 24 hours. From purulent or semi-purulent exudates, from glands or from the lungs cultivations in broth or on agar are usually sufficient. Small pieces of the gland or of the lung-tissue, the exposed surface of which has been well seared, should be cut out with a sterile knife or scissors and the portion put at once into the fluid medium or crushed and rubbed over the surface of the solid medium.

For staining the films, methylene blue, thionin blue or carbol-fuchsin should be employed. It may be necessary, where organisms of the diphtheroid type are found, to use special stains, and even to inoculate animals, but for details of these methods of examination reference must be made to text-books of bacteriology. Where tuberculosis is suspected, but is not definite enough to be diagnosed by naked eye examination, scrapings from the suspected area should be stained by the Ziehl-Neelsen method and examined for *B. tuberculosis*, or sections should be made and examined for giant-cells or other histological structure of tubercle or an emulsion of the suspected tissue should be inoculated into a guinea-pig.

TYPHOID FEVER.

The external examination, the opening of the body and the removal of the organs are carried out precisely in the manner described for general post-mortems, though it is generally useful to remove the intestines before the other viscera. Great care should be exercised in this removal lest the bowel be torn and artificial lacerations mistaken for perforations. Perforation should be carefully looked for, and any localised deposits of lymph which might be sealing up actual holes in the bowel should be carefully examined. The whole extent of the bowels, but especially the small intestine, the cæcum and the colon on their mucous surfaces, should be examined for swelling of and ulceration in the Peyer's patches and the solitary glands, and the presence of swelling, of sloughs and of ulceration carefully noted. It is usually of very little value to attempt cultivations of B. *typhosus* from the ulcers, as the organism can be more readily recovered from the spleen.

The general characters of the spleen are noted, especially its firm consistence which distinguishes it from the spleen in most of the other acute infective fevers. For bacteriological examination the surface of the organ should be seared, the capsule cut through with a sterile knife and the pulp torn by folding the spleen either in its transverse or its long axis.

A small quantity of the pulp should be scraped from various areas with a spoon-shaped platinum needle or with a sterilised knife, or small portions should be excised at several places and crushed, and this material inoculated either in a series of broth tubes, on agar plates, or on plates or tubes containing such special media as McConkey's bile-salt-lactose, etc. *Infarct* and *gangrenous abscesses* may be found in the spleen and special bacteriological examination should be made of such areas.

The liver may shew cloudy swelling and small areas of necrosis, and similar conditions may be found in the kidneys and in the mesenteric glands. Suppurative foci are sometimes found in the kidneys and in the mesenteric glands, and such foci must be examined bacteriologically. Careful search should always be made in the larynx for ulceration, the sites of election being the posterior wall at the insertion of the cords, the base of the epiglottis and the ary-epiglottic fold. The cartilages may become inflamed and necrosed. Lobar and catarrhal pneumonia may be present, while gangrene of the lung, pleurisy and hæmorrhagic infarction are less common.

In the heart endocarditis, pericarditis and myocarditis may be found and an arteritis with thrombosis has been described. Thrombosis of the veins, especially of the left femoral, is more common.

The muscles, especially of the abdominal wall, should be carefully examined for any evidence of Zenker's degeneration, which may also, however, occur in the adductors of the thigh and in the pectorals.

The gall bladder should be carefully searched for any catarrhal condition and culture tubes inoculated, not only from the bile, but also from scrapings from the mucous membrane of the bladder.

Any nervous manifestations will call for special examination of the brain and cord for meningitis, encephalitis, hæmorrhage, etc.

Abscesses in the bones with periostitis, necrosis or caries should be looked for.

Bacteriological examination. As already stated the spleen and the gall bladder should always be examined for the presence of *B. typhosus*, and all suppurative, ulcerative or necrotic foci should, in like manner, be examined to determine, if possible, whether these pathological conditions are due to *B. typhosus*, to some of the pyogenetic organisms, or to an association of the latter with *B. typhosus*. The urine should be examined by cultural methods to determine the presence or absence of *B. typhosus*. Full details of the methods for isolation of *B. typhosus* will be found in text-books of bacteriology. Suffice it to say here that the preliminary cultures should be made on ordinary slant agar tubes or on plates of agar containing dextrose, lactose, bile salts, neutral red, etc.

In any doubtful case some blood should be reserved in capillary tubes for agglutination reactions.

Film preparations from suppurative foci, etc. are not of much value for diagnostic purposes, but they may help in the determination of further procedure.

PLAGUE.

In examining cases suspected to be plague a careful search must be made for any enlarged glands, and the lungs should also be carefully examined for any signs of pneumonia, but histological and bacteriological examination are alone of any value in diagnosis.

Scrapings from the suspected glands, from the spleen, from the lungs or from the bronchial secretions, filmed on glass slides, and stained with any of the aniline dyes, preferably thionin blue, are usually sufficient for diagnosis—the typical organisms, shewing their bipolar staining, being very abundant. I have, however, seen films from pneumonic sputum, in which organisms morphologically identical with B. pestis were abundant, and from cases where there was no reason to suspect plague. It is therefore important that microscopical examination of films should be followed by attempts to cultivate the organism. Cultures should be made from the heart-blood, from the spleen, suspected glands, lungs, etc. The outer surface of the glands or spleen, or of the pneumonic area in the lungs, should be carefully seared, small pieces of tissue cut out, crushed between sterile glass plates and inoculated into some of the ordinary media—agar or broth—the agar preferably in plates, in order that separation from other associated organisms may be effected. Suspicious colonies are examined microscopically in smear preparations.

If doubt still exists, rats or mice, which are extremely susceptible, should be inoculated and, after death, scrapings made from their spleen and cultures from the heart-blood.

The pathologist may be called upon to examine rats suspected to be carriers of B. pestis. Before commencing the examination the rat should be dipped in some solution which will destroy any fleas which may be present and which might spread the infection. The Port Sanitary Authorities of Liverpool have all rats dipped in petrol before they are sent for examination. Rats coming from other authorities are treated with a fairly strong solution of lysol. An incision is made along the ventral surface from pelvis to jaw, and the skin, etc. pulled outwards so that glands in the neck, in the axilla and in the groin are exposed, and the liver, spleen and lungs brought into view.

Subcutaneous congestion, particularly in the region of the bubo, is looked for, as it is not infrequently a well-marked feature. This congestion gives to the muscles a purplish-pink colour, which should always arouse suspicion.

Subcutaneous hæmorrhages, particularly in the submaxillary region, are frequently seen, and these are usually in the neighbourhood of buboes. The Advisory Committee, in their Plague Investigations in India, state that they have never observed these hæmorrhages in any rat which was not plague-infected.

Enlarged glands. In septicæmic cases the glands in any region of the body may be enlarged and congested, and in the bubonic form there may be primary enlargement in one area with secondary involvement of the glands in other regions. These primary or secondary buboes may shew points of hæmorrhage when cut across, and there may be considerable infiltration, with, perhaps, hæmorrhage in the subcutaneous tissues in the neighbourhood of the bubo. This condition is usually most marked round primary buboes. The most common situation for the enlarged glands in the rat is in the submaxillary region, though they may be found in the groin and in the axilla. Any enlarged gland should be cut into, and if there is any evidence of necrosis this area should be most carefully examined.

The liver. The liver becomes congested and fatty, and presents a "mottled" appearance—the pink congested areas contrasting with the yellow fatty ones   Sometimes the degree of fatty degeneration is very marked—the whole liver being smooth and yellowish in colour. Yellowish or greyish necrotic patches are also seen.   These various degrees of fatty degeneration are in my experience fairly common in rats, and I am not inclined to attach too much weight to this "mottling" in the diagnosis of plague.

The spleen. The spleen is often somewhat enlarged and is always firm in consistence, and sometimes presents a slightly granular surface.

There are no specially characteristic features in the other

organs, except that clear serous effusion occurs in quite a number of cases in plague-infected rats.

Thus " the most important post-mortem features for purposes of diagnosis " are, according to the reports on " Plague investigation in India " of the Advisory Committee appointed by the Secretary of State for India, the Royal Society and the Lister Institute :

(*a*) The presence of a typical bubo.
(*b*) The " granular " or mottled liver.
(*c*) Subcutaneous hæmorrhages.
(*d*) An abundant clear pleural effusion.

The absence of all these signs is of great importance, but the presence of even one of them makes it imperative that a careful bacteriological examination both by microscopical, cultural and inoculation methods should be carried out.

Influenza and Cerebro-spinal Meningitis.

Neither of these diseases requires any modification from the ordinary procedure. In both the lungs should be carefully examined for pneumonia and for pleurisy, and bacteriological examination made of any purulent exudate. In influenza the nasal and the bronchial secretion should be carefully searched by film methods and by culture for the causal bacillus. The influenza bacillus is best grown both in primary and in subculture on blood agar, and it is frequently associated with pneumococcus and other organisms. The meningococcus often presents great difficulty in cultivation and the pus should be inoculated on to a blood serum mixture directly from the exudate and as early as possible. Film preparations are valuable in the diagnosis of the meningococcus in pus.

The differentiation of the influenza bacillus and of the meningococcus from allied organisms or similar morphological characters is usually not difficult, but for the methods of doing this the reader is referred to special works on bacteriology.

SMALL-POX.

The larynx should always be examined for evidence of inflammation and involvement of the cartilages. The lungs may shew congestion or broncho-pneumonia and in the heart myocarditis may occur. In the hæmorrhagic form, numerous areas of hæmorrhage may be found in the serous and mucous surfaces, in the parenchyma of the various organs, in the connective tissue and in the sheaths of the nerves. The spleen is usually enlarged and the liver fatty. These changes should be specially looked for, but otherwise the post-mortem examination should be done in the ordinary way.

WHOOPING COUGH.

No special directions need be given for a post-mortem in a case of whooping cough. Broncho-pneumonia with collapse and areas of emphysema are usually found. Bacteriological examination of the secretion in the bronchi should be made for any organisms and especially for the Bordet-Gengou bacillus. This can be grown on 1 % glycerine agar, or in broth made with macerated potato, to which is added an equal volume of human or rabbit blood. Some blood should be taken for testing the agglutination and the complement deviation reactions.

CHOLERA AND DYSENTERY.

In both these diseases the pathologist will give special attention to the intestine. In cholera he will find the mucous membrane of the small intestine swollen and hyperæmic and the epithelium denuded, but usually there is no evidence of ulceration; in dysentery the ulceration is a marked feature, and is usually confined to the large intestine and the lower portion of the ileum. The ulcers are usually irregular in outline with infiltrated and undermined edges. In cholera the walls of the intestine are thinned, whereas in dysentery they are much thickened, owing to an infiltration of the submucous tissues with inflammatory products.

In cholera, there may be an intense colitis with a membranous deposit, and a similar membranous deposit may be seen in other severe forms of colitis or entero-colitis where there has been necrosis of the mucous membrane. It is often difficult to clearly differentiate these cases from dysentery.

In dysentery, abscess of the liver should always be looked for, and any evidence of communication between the abscess and the right lung. Pneumonia and pleurisy may occur in cases of cholera, but these conditions are not in any way characteristic.

Bacteriological examination of the fæces in all suspected cases of cholera should be undertaken. McLaughlin recommends that 1 gram of the fæces should be added to 100 c.c. of sterile peptone solution (*vide* Appendix) and incubated for 6 hours at 35 to 37° C. Smears from the surface film should then be made, stained with carbol-fuchsin and examined carefully for any suspicious organisms. If organisms are found, plates are made and detailed examination is then proceeded with.

The stools or the ulcerated patches in the intestine must also be examined for *B. dysenteria*. Kendall and Walker give the following method as the most useful.

" After plating on Endo's medium (see Appendix) small translucent colonies are transferred to mannite-litmus semi-solid media and incubated for twenty-four hours. Non-spreading growths in the medium are then examined further for agglutinative and other characteristics. The mannite furnishes a means of differentiating between the Shiga (non-mannite, fermenting) and Flexner (mannite, fermenting) types of dysentery bacillus Acid, but no gas, is formed in the medium, whereas *B. coli*, *B. cloacæ*, and *B. proteus*, which are common in the intestine, form gas. Agglutination with specific serum must be the final test."

The amœba of dysentery may be found on microscopical examination in the intestinal contents or in the mucous membrane. If a liver-abscess is present the amœba may be found in scrapings from the wall, though it may be absent in the necrotic contents of the abscess.

YELLOW FEVER.

The post-mortem examination is carried out by the routine procedure already described, but the liver is specially examined for fatty degeneration and areas of necrosis. Fatty and necrotic changes are also found in the kidneys and less intensely in the muscle of the heart. Some observers regard the extreme fatty and necrotic changes in the liver as characteristic.

BERI-BERI.

The only constant features in beri-beri which call for special examination are the degenerative and inflammatory changes which affect the axis cylinders and the medullary sheaths of the peripheral nerves. Occasionally the pneumogastric and the phrenic nerves are involved.

MALTA FEVER.

In fatal cases, which are comparatively rare, there are no special characteristic morbid changes. Cultures should be made from the spleen and sufficient blood should be taken for agglutination tests.

PUERPERAL FEVER—RHEUMATIC FEVER.

These diseases may involve a prolonged post-mortem examination, but the method of procedure is the general one which has been described.

Bacteriological examination must be made of any secretion or exudate and in rheumatic fever of any vegetations and of the synovial membranes from affected joints. I have already described in Chapter IX the method of procedure in regard to joints.

TETANUS.

The wound, if it has not been excised, should be examined bacteriologically. There are no morbid appearances which are characteristic of the disease in any of the organs, and therefore a post-mortem examination is of little value. There may be indefinite patches of softening in the grey matter of the cord, medulla and pons. The nerve trunks leading from the original area of infection may shew a marked neuritis. There may be signs of laceration and bruising of the muscle fibres in various parts of the body.

For bacteriological examination the excised wound, or scrapings from it, should be inoculated in a glucose broth media and incubated anærobically and after spore formation has taken place, the non-sporing organisms killed by exposure to a temperature of about 80° C.

ANTHRAX.

1. *Malignant pustule.* The death in such cases is usually due to septicæmia and there may be no special pathological changes in any of the internal organs or tissues. The blood should be examined for *B. anthracis.* In some cases enteritis, peritonitis, endocarditis and hæmorrhagic meningitis have been described and these conditions therefore should be borne in mind in all cases.

2. *Woolsorters' disease.* Special examination is made of the lower part of the trachea and the upper part of the large bronchi for evidences of swelling, hæmorrhage and œdema. The mediastinal and the bronchial glands may be enormously enlarged, there may be pleural and pericardial effusion and the lungs may shew congestion, œdema and collapse.

3. *Intestinal anthrax.* The mucous membrane of the intestine may shew intense inflammation with hæmorrhage and necrosis.

Bacteriological examination. Whatever the lesion present, the blood, and the hæmorrhagic and the necrotic areas, especially at their peripheries, should be examined by film and culture for *B. anthracis.* It is extremely important that this examination should be exhaustive as some of the organisms found in putrefactive areas resemble in morphology and even in cultural characters *B. anthracis.*

GLANDERS.

In dealing with a case of glanders the pathologist must always remember that the glands in connection with the local lesion may suppurate and that pyæmic abscesses may occur in the lungs, the spleen, the liver, the bone marrow and the salivary glands, or that the local lesion may form an ulcer with thickened margins and spreading deeply into the tissues, that the thickened lymphatic channels may ulcerate and that areas of necrotic granulation tissue may be found in the subcutaneous tissues, in the muscles and in the mucous membranes. Films from the pus or scrapings from the necrotic tissue may reveal the causal organism, which however stains rather feebly with the aniline dyes unless the staining process is prolonged for 15 to 30 minutes Cultures, however, should always be made on a nutrient agar and on potato. Emulsions of the cultures or of the pus or necrotic tissue should for diagnostic purposes be inoculated in the peritoneal cavity of a male guinea-pig. The testicles shew marked swelling with central necrosis in from three to four days.

HYDROPHOBIA OR RABIES.

The post-mortem examination is done in the usual way, and little information is got except from examination of the sections or scrapings from the brain. There is still much uncertainty as to whether any of the lesions which have been found and described as characteristic by various authors are really pathognomonic of the disease. An accumulation of leucocytes around the blood vessels and the nerve cells, particularly the motor ganglion cells, of the central nervous system has been described, but this may occur in other diseases. Again van Gehuchten and Nelis attributed considerable importance to the accumulation of lymphoid and endothelial cells around nerve cells of the sympathetic and cerebro-spinal ganglia. Negri described round, oval or angular bodies which, stained by Giemsa's process, were pale blue in colour and contained certain round or oval pink bodies and some smaller red or violet-red granules. These "Negri bodies" found in the large nerve cells of the central nervous system are regarded by many as protozoal in nature and as specific of hydrophobia, and therefore, in the examination of any case of this nature, these bodies should be searched for.

The pathologist may have to settle the diagnosis in any given case, and for this purpose two methods are employed :

1. Smears or sections are made from the brain, by preference from the hippocampus, and search is made for Negri bodies.

The hippocampus is seen as a laterally arched ridge forming the floor of the lateral ventricle, and is exposed by removing horizontal slices of the brain until the lateral ventricle is reached and then removing the roof of the ventricle. The smears may be stained by Giemsa's stain for from half-an-hour to three hours ; the preparation being then washed and dried.

The bodies stain deeply with the eosin part of the stain, while the granules take on the blue of the methylene blue.

Sections may be fixed in Zenker's solution, embedded in paraffin, cut and stained with eosin and methylene blue, or with iron hæmatoxylin.

2. A small quantity (1 or 2 c.c.) of the medulla or cord of the suspected case is rubbed up in a sterile mortar with about 10 c.c. of sterile distilled water, and the solution filtered through ordinary filter paper to remove tissue-shreds. A few drops of the fluid thus obtained are injected between the dura mater and the surface of the brain of a rabbit. The skin over the anterior part of the cranium is painted with iodine or sterilised in some other way, and an incision made through the skin in the middle line between the eyes. Then with a small trephine, or the blade of a pair of sharp-pointed scissors, or with a special boring instrument, similar to the one illustrated on p. 166, an opening is made in the skull in the median line at a point just posterior to a line drawn through the middle of each eye. The fluid is drawn up into a piece of glass tubing bent at an obtuse angle, the narrow end of the tube is introduced carefully between the dura mater and the brain, and the fluid is gently blown or pressed by means of a rubber teat into the subdural

space. The wound in the scalp is now carefully closed—the whole operation should be done with strict aseptic precautions and with the animal anæsthetised.

The symptoms of experimental rabies are exhibited by weakness of the hind limbs followed by paralysis, which soon extends to the fore limbs, the rabbit dying with marked dyspnœa about three days after the onset of the first symptoms.

The early symptoms do not appear till at least 14 days after the inoculation, and they may not appear until one or two months. The early paralyses which may follow injury to the brain during the operation or the later results of sepsis are not likely to be mistaken for hydrophobic symptoms, if the operator bears in mind the late onset of the rabic paralysis. In negative cases it is my practice to give a preliminary report one month after inoculation, and a final report in two months.

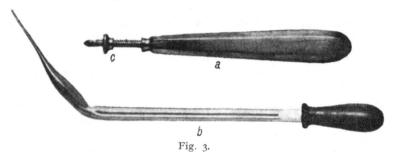

Fig. 3.

a. Boring instrument for skull. *c.* Screw for regulating depth of penetration.
b. Glass tube for introducing fluid under the dura—the upper end is plugged with cotton wool.

SYPHILIS.

In cases of syphilis or supposed syphilis, the lesions to be specially searched for will depend upon the stage of the disease ; but the majority of cases which come to the post-mortem room are of the tertiary type, and to this I shall confine the examination.

A preliminary inspection should be made for evidence of the lesions, or the scars of the lesions, of the earlier stages— such as chancres about the penis, the labia, the rectum, the lips, etc., the presence of periosteal nodes about the bones, particularly the tibiæ, ulcerated patches, and mucous patches or condylomata.

In congenital cases, note should be made of the condition of the teeth, the presence of depression of the bridge of the nose, keratitis or iritis, necrotic patches on the bones of the skull, periosteal nodes, joint lesions, etc.

In the more advanced and tertiary cases, the bones, especially those of the skull, should be examined for periostitis and necrosis. Perforations of the palate and of the larynx are sometimes found.

Brain and spinal cord. Meningitis, giving rise to localised thickening of the membranes, often with compression of the cranial nerves near their orifices of exit, is sometimes present. Gummata at these spots should be carefully looked for, though gummata may also be found without this evidence of meningitis.

Areas of softening and sclerosis should always be looked for, both in the brain and the spinal cord. The softening is usually easily detected, and is commonly due to arterial degeneration with thrombosis, or to the obstruction of the blood supply by the pressure and infiltration of gummata ; the latter condition is best examined microscopically.

Lungs. Three main conditions call for special attention.

1. *White pneumonia* which occurs in the fœtus and is very commonly associated with scattered miliary white foci which are specially seen round the arteries.

2. *Gummata* These may vary considerably in size and are found particularly towards the root of the lungs, and from them white strands of fibrous tissue are often seen radiating into the lung substance.

3. *White bands of fibrous tissue* may produce a well-marked interstitial pneumonia, particularly in the lower lobes and near the root. The outer surface of the lung may exhibit very irregular scarring as a result of the contraction of this fibrous tissue.

Larynx. There may be deep, irregular ulceration and extensive infiltration of the whole of the tissues of the larynx. Irregular contractions and partial stenosis may be produced by cicatrisation. The ulcers should be specially looked for at the upper part of the larynx in the region of the vocal cords, but they may be found in other places and the trachea and larger bronchi may become involved secondarily. Perichondritis, especially of the cricoid cartilage, should be looked for. *Heart.* Gummata sometimes occur and may be widely spread in the septum ventriculorum or elsewhere. They are always associated with very considerable fibrosis.

Arteries. Degenerative (arterio-sclerotic and atheromatous) changes are generally quite obvious to the naked eye, but in the smaller vessels only microscopical examination will shew the exact nature of the changes.

Liver. Diffuse syphilitic hepatitis, such as is seen in congenital cases, may not present any very obvious naked eye changes, though the liver may be somewhat enlarged and firmer than normal. Strands of connective tissue may sometimes be seen separating the liver cells into small groups. Irregular scarring of the liver may be present only to a slight degree or may be so pronounced as to divide the tissue up into small and irregular lobules. On section fibrous bands may be seen cutting up the liver substance into larger or smaller irregular areas, and gummata are frequently present. Perihepatitis with considerable thickening of Glisson's capsule is sometimes associated with syphilis.

Digestive tract. Ulcers and stenosis should be looked for in the œsophagus and intestine. The most common site for stenosis is the rectum and this is usually due to gummatous infiltration of the submucosa just above the internal sphincter.

Kidneys. Acute syphilitic nephritis may occur, but is not in any way specific in its naked eye or microscopical characters, but chronic interstitial nephritis is common.

Testicles. Gummatous infiltration and interstitial fibrosis of the testicles should always be looked for in cases of syphilis.

In the earlier stages of the disease scrapings should be taken from chancres, ulcerated patches, etc., and in the later stages sections may be made which, together with any fluids found, should be examined for *spirochæta pallida*.

Amyloid degeneration should always be examined for in the liver, spleen, kidneys and lymphatic glands.

In obscure cases where syphilis is suspected, cerebro-spinal fluid or blood should be collected in order that a Wassermann reaction should be tried, if this has not already been done during life.

TUBERCULOSIS.

In examining cadavers it must always be borne in mind that tuberculosis may be a secondary process, and the real cause of the condition from which the patient has died may be quite independent of the tuberculous lesion, or, on the other hand, the important lesion for investigation may be non-tuberculous though the death was due to the secondary tuberculosis. Thus in examining the lungs of grinders the fibrosis is the more important condition, though in the majority of cases the death is due to tuberculosis, or again, cases of lymphadenoma may be complicated by tuberculosis and the really important lesion obscured if the tuberculous process is far advanced.

On the other hand, small localised tuberculous foci are either missed or thought to be so unimportant that no note is made of them. I cannot too strongly urge all pathologists to carefully note all such lesions however small or apparently unimportant they may seem to be at the time of the examination. The areas which should be specially examined in such cases are the mesenteric glands, the apices and the roots of the lungs, and the glands about the angles of the jaws.

In cases in which the mesenteric glands are affected the intestines should be examined for any evidence of ulceration.

Where the kidneys are affected the ureters, the bladder, the vas deferens and the epididymis and testicle should be examined, if there is any reason to suspect that the condition is not localised to the kidneys.

General miliary tuberculosis is always so easily recognised that little need be said except that a careful search should be made for any special focus which may have been the starting point for the general infection—such for example as a mesenteric gland, an old nodule at the apex of the lung, or a mass in bone. In many cases it may not be possible to trace such primary foci.

Localised miliary tuberculosis. Miliary tuberculosis localised to a single organ is rare except in the lungs, but the condition may be simulated by minute areas of necrosis in the liver, by infiltration of the liver, spleen or kidney with leucocytes in leucocythæmia, especially in the lymphatic type of the disease, and by lymphadenomatous nodules in the spleen. Swollen Malpighian bodies in the spleen are sometimes mistaken for tubercle granulations. I have seen a case of minute abscesses in the lungs, due to one of the *streptothriciæ*, which resembled very closely acute miliary tuberculosis. If there is the least doubt, in any given case, histological examination should be made.

Tuberculosis in the lungs. The examination does not involve the adoption of any special method, but a careful description of all cavities should be made—their exact site, the character of their walls and their contents, and, if possible, whether they definitely communicate with bronchi. The larynx and trachea should be carefully examined for any evidence of tuberculous infiltration or ulceration. It is desirable in many cases to make a bacteriological examination of the contents of the cavities for organisms other than *B. tuberculosis*.

Tuberculosis of the larynx. Careful examination should be made for :

1. Minute, shallow ulcers, especially near the margins of the vocal cords and on the posterior commissure.

2. Extensive tubercular infiltration, especially of the ary-epiglottic folds and of the epiglottis itself.

3. Perichondritis, especially to the arytenoid and the thyroid cartilages.

Tuberculosis of the intestines. The intestines should always be opened in the ordinary way in cases of tuberculosis, and careful search made for ulcers and these accurately described, and any evidence of stenosis noted.

Tuberculosis in the other thoracic or abdominal organs does not demand any special method of examination and the only point that need be mentioned is that care should be taken not to confuse the lesions with syphilitic gummata, lymphadenoma, leucocythæmia, or with abscess formation. Histological examination will clear up any doubt.

Tuberculosis of the brain and spinal cord. In all cases of tuberculosis of the brain, the spinal cord should also be examined. The small tubercle granulations on the meninges may sometimes be difficult to see with the naked eye, even in the Sylvian fissures where they are usually prominent, but, if a portion of the membrane is spread on a slide, microscopical examination with a low power will reveal the granulations. Warning has already been given not to confuse the Pacchionian bodies with tubercle granulations. In cases of tuberculous meningitis, the brain, and particularly the cerebellum and pons, should be examined for so-called tuberculous tumours.

Sleeping Sickness.

The post-mortem examination should be conducted in the ordinary way, but the pathologist should be careful to collect as much cerebro-spinal fluid as possible in order to search for trypanosomes, and he should remove some of the enlarged glands, which are always a striking feature at the post-mortem examination, and examine the pulp of these for trypanosomes.

There are no other specially characteristic features noticeable at the post-mortem ; the brain usually shews a chronic meningo-encephalitis with excess of fluid in the subarachnoid space. This fluid is sometimes turbid but rarely purulent. The heart may shew myocardial changes, and there may be patches of broncho-pneumonia in both lungs.

Portions of the brain with its membranes, particularly at the base, and of the spinal cord should be removed for subsequent examination. Mott has described a marked infiltration of mononuclear leucocytes in the pia-arachnoid, a perivascular infiltration of the same type of cell in the substance of the brain and various pathological changes in the nerve-cells—in the axis cylinders and in the medullary sheaths.

An examination of the vessels of the brain and cord for endarteritis is important, for in some cases simulating sleeping sickness tumours of the brain especially of syphilitic origin have been found, and in these cases the syphilitic endarteritis is present—in sleeping sickness endarteritis is not present.

Syphilis may also produce the meningo-encephalitis seen in sleeping sickness, and in general paralysis of the insane the symptoms may resemble those of sleeping sickness. It is therefore important not only to search for the trypanosomes but also to examine for the *spirochæta pallida* in doubtful cases.

KALA-AZAR.

As the post-mortem diagnosis depends on the finding of the Leishman-Donovan bodies the cases usually present no difficulty to the pathologist. It is however interesting if not important that his examination for the parasites should not be confined to one organ   In the spleen, which is usually much enlarged, they are present in enormous numbers, and film preparations from the pulp, stained by Leishman's or Giemsa's method, are quite sufficient to establish the diagnosis.

The liver may also be enlarged and shew signs of chronic congestion and the cells containing parasites are seen in large numbers, either free or partially attached to the walls of the dilated intralobular capillaries.   Cirrhosis and fatty degeneration should be looked for as these conditions have been described in association with kala-azar, though the causal relationship of the cirrhosis is, to say the least, doubtful.

The bone marrow should be examined by film-preparations as it is very often very heavily infected.

Ulcers in the skin and ulcers in the intestine should be very carefully looked for.   The intestinal ulcers are most commonly found in the colon and the sigmoid flexure, and in many cases these may be dysenteric in origin, but apparently they may occur as a definite lesion in kala-azar.   The mesenteric glands are often intensely infected, especially if they drain an ulcerated area.

The other organs shew no special changes though parasites may be found in the kidneys, the suprarenal glands, the pancreas, the testicles and the lungs.

MALARIA AND BLACKWATER FEVER.

These diseases which are intimately associated present no difficulties as to the methods of performing the post-mortem examination, but it is important to examine carefully in both diseases for evidence of malarial pigmentation and parasites in the blood and in the various organs.

The fatal cases of malaria are usually of the malignant type and though the parasites may be scanty in the general circulation, they may be found in considerable numbers in certain organs, particularly the spleen and the bone-marrow. They may also be found in the brain forming with the pigment actual thrombi in the small vessels.

The spleen and the liver should always be examined for necrotic areas, and the liver for cirrhosis.

In blackwater fever malarial parasites are very commonly absent in the internal organs, though they have been found in the brain. Malarial pigment is found in the spleen and in the liver, necrotic areas and thrombi are found in the liver, the kidneys usually shew no melanin, and the only important change is degeneration of the epithelium lining the convoluted tubules.

SPRUE.

In examining such cases the pathologist must specially direct his attention to the intestinal canal, examining it from mouth to anus and observing any evidence of congestion, erosion, ulceration and cicatrisation. The mesenteric glands may shew enlargement and fibrosis. Mucous cysts are very common in the intestine and are probably due to obstruction in the follicles. The other organs must of course be carefully examined, but they generally shew no characteristic changes. Tuberculosis is not uncommon in the lungs.

LEPROSY.

Systematic examination must be made for " leprous nodules " in the skin, in the mucous membranes of the mouth and throat, in the nerve trunks, in the lymphatic glands, in the testes and in the liver. The other internal organs do not usually shew special changes, though the bacilli may be present in enormous numbers. Under the microscope the nodules are seen to be very cellular, though fibrous transformation may be seen at parts and " lepra " cells may be present in large or small numbers. The diagnosis depends on the finding of the characteristic bacillus in these nodules.

Scrapings are taken from the nodules, the material spread on slides and stained with carbol-fuchsin as for *B. tuberculosis*— the decolourisation however being carried out with 5 % sulphuric acid and the acid acting for about one minute.

Tuberculosis is very commonly associated with leprosy, and it is therefore important to differentiate the two organisms which are both of the acid-fast type—the bacillus of leprosy is however easily decolourised with weak (5 %) sulphuric acid.

Chronic renal disease is also common ; and search should always be made for septic foci in the viscera. Amyloid degeneration has been described and should be looked for. The spinal cord should be examined for sclerotic changes, though in many cases the cord appears to be quite healthy.

Yaws, Delhi Boil, Tropical Skin Diseases other than those due to Tuberculosis and Syphilis.

The pathological lesions associated with these diseases are usually examined during life, and there are no distinctive post-mortem appearances.

The various nodules, ulcerated areas, etc., are examined by scrapings or films and by microscopical sections for parasites which are supposed to be causal. The methods to be followed are not in any way special and need not be described. Films are prepared and stained by Giemsa's or Leishman's method.

In yaws, *spirochæta* have to be looked for in the manner described under syphilis ; in Delhi boil, protozoa resembling, if not identical with Leishman-Donovan bodies ; and in skin diseases, fungi, bacteria, protozoa, etc. Care must always be taken to differentiate these conditions from tuberculosis and syphilis.

DISEASES IN THE THORACIC ORGANS.

By following closely the method of examination already described for the thoracic organs no important pathological condition is likely to be missed. I would however again emphasise the very great importance of the careful examination of the vessels of the heart for degenerative changes and for thrombosis, and the vessels of the lungs for thrombi or for emboli.

Small necrotic areas in the heart (*myomalacia cordis*) are very apt to be missed, especially when they occur towards the posterior surface, and if the vessels are found to be degenerated in any marked degree these areas should be specially looked for.

Thrombi or emboli in the vessels of the lungs are generally evidenced by the presence of infarcts, but cases occur not infrequently without any apparent gross lesion.

Endocarditis and Myocarditis.

In examining cases of endocarditis or acute myocarditis I have found it advantageous, especially in rheumatic cases, to make cultivations in the special media recommended by Poynton and Paine—equal parts of milk and nutrient broth slightly acidified with a 10 % solution of lactic acid. Cultures however should also be made on blood agar for *pneumococci*, for *B. influenza*, etc.

In cases with a history of rheumatic fever search should be made for rheumatic nodules in the heart, and in all cases it is advisable to have the muscle-substance examined microscopically at various areas, even though no pathological change is evident to the naked eye.

Pneumonia.

In all types of this disease bacteriological examination should be made not only of the lung itself but also of the blood from the heart. In cases which are caused by the *pneumococcus* or *B. pestis* the best procedure is direct inoculation of the blood or of an emulsion of the lung substance in saline into mice, though cultures should also be made on agar or blood agar. It should always be remembered that the *pneumococcus* may have become enfeebled and that the mouse does not necessarily die as a result of the inoculation though the organisms may be present in considerable numbers. The *pneumococcus* or *B. pestis* may be associated with other organisms, and cultures are necessary in order to determine this point, for in the inoculated animals the infection by *pneumococcus* or *B. pestis* may be so pronounced that the associated organisms are completely lost, and it may be important in any given case to determine the relation of these organisms to the disease.

Thus in cases of typhoid fever, where secondary pneumonia develops, it may be very important to determine whether the *pneumococcus*, which is so often found, is the primary cause of the pneumonia or only a secondary invader. The death of a mouse from pneumococcal septicæmia in such cases is often taken as proof that the lung condition is really pneumococcal in origin—a position which in my opinion is quite unjustifiable.

In all cases of pneumonia the pericardium and epicardium should be carefully examined for any evidence of pericarditis, and special attention should be directed to the base of the heart round the great vessels and also on the posterior surface. It should also be borne in mind that peritonitis and meningitis may be associated with pneumonia.

Empyema.

Bacteriological examination of the pus should be made in all cases. Occasionally the pus is sterile, due to the destruction of the organisms. I have found in some of these cases, which have been secondary to pneumonia, that though it was difficult to demonstrate the bacteria with the ordinary staining methods, the capsules could be made out when special " capsule stains " were used, and the causal organisms in two or three cases have been clearly demonstrated in this way.

Bronchiectasis.

I have elsewhere emphasised the importance of making a careful bacteriological examination of the secretions which are found in dilated bronchiectatic cavities, and, in cases of meningitis or of cerebral abscess, in septicæmia or pyæmia, where the cause is not clear, it is always advisable to examine the lungs carefully for small localised dilatations of the bronchi, in which secretions have accumulated and undergone septic transformation. In a few cases of meningitis, I have found the primary infective area in such cavities and have been able to isolate *streptococcus pyogenes* from the cavity and from the pus on the surface of the brain.

Bronchitis.

Acute catarrhal bronchitis. At a post-mortem examination acute catarrhal bronchitis is rarely found unassociated with other pulmonary conditions and is particularly associated with broncho-pneumonia and with emphysema. It may be a complication of pulmonary tuberculosis, interstitial pneumonia, etc. In typical acute cases, the mucous membrane of the trachea and bronchi is reddened, congested and covered with mucus and muco-pus and, when pressure is exerted on the lung, pus may be seen oozing from the smaller bronchi, some of which are seen to be dilated.

Chronic bronchitis. The appearances vary considerably but usually the secretion is very abundant and definitely purulent. The mucous membrane may shew a brownish-red or slaty-blue pigmentation, and the lumen of the bronchi may be dilated. It is always well to search for small ulcerated areas between the rings of cartilage. These are specially seen in the more advanced stages of the disease when the mucous membrane becomes thinned and atrophied and the longitudinal bands of elastic tissue stand out prominently.

Membranous or plastic bronchitis (Fibrinous bronchitis). Whitish or greyish-white casts or remains of these may be found in the bronchial passages, and the bronchial mucous membrane may be injected or pale. Emphysema is almost invariably present. The casts must always be examined very carefully to exclude the possibility of their being diphtheritic in origin.

Collapse and Atelectasis.

These conditions are very similar in their general appearances and it may be necessary to differentiate carefully between the two. Collapse is very much commoner and the associated lesions found at the post-mortem examination usually leave no doubt as to the condition. In both, the affected area of the lung is much reduced in size, is depressed below the general level, is often of a slaty-bluish or purplish colour, and is extremely tough and resistant. Bronchial dilatation may be present, and the pleura over the collapsed area may or may not be thickened. In true atelectasis, at any rate when seen in the newly born, the collapsed part can be inflated from the corresponding bronchi; but if the patient lives for some time fibrous tissue overgrowth may take place, and an actual obliteration of the lung alveoli may occur. In these cases the affected lung tissue is usually pale and characterised by a great deficiency of carbon pigment as compared with the opposite lung or the unaffected part of the same lung, and the bronchi frequently shew marked dilatation.

Lobular collapse is very frequent as a result of capillary bronchitis, especially in young children.

Chronic Interstitial Pneumonia.

The fibrosed areas may be small and scattered, the overgrowth of fibrous tissue may follow the lines of the interlobular septa, producing a reticulated appearance in the lungs, or almost the whole lung may be fibrosed. In all cases particular note should be made of the condition of the pleura, as to general thickening or the presence of small pearl-like areas of fibrous tissue which are always very apparent in the lungs of stone-hewers and grinders. These areas are usually surrounded by a zone of pigmentation. Special attention should be directed to the lower lobes towards the posterior aspect, as I have sometimes found localised areas of fibrosis at this situation.

In all cases it is important to search carefully for evidence of tuberculosis. This is commonly very apparent, but in some cases, *e.g.* from the Sheffield grinders, the evidence of tubercular infection was very slight, and might easily be overlooked. There seems little doubt that fibrosed lungs are very liable to be infected by *B. tuberculosis*, but the spread of the tuberculous process in them may be slow.

The pulmonary arteries should always be examined as atheromatous changes are common. Dilatation of bronchi is always present and may be excessive in amount, producing a series of bronchiectatic cavities. Endarteritis of the syphilitic type should always be looked for, especially in cases of fibrosis of the lower lobes where there is no definite evidence of the inhalation of foreign, irritating particles, and, where scarring of the lobe is seen, search should be made for gummata or other new growth.

Mediastinal Growths.

Usually these present no special difficulties at a post-mortem examination. In dealing with them I have always found it advisable to remove the whole of the thoracic contents with the trachea and larynx, the œsophagus having been previously tied just above the diaphragm. The mass which has been removed should now be carefully examined and note specially made of any displacement of, or pressure upon, the œsophagus, the aorta, the trachea and bronchi and the larger veins. The œsophagus, the aorta and its branches, the trachea and the larger bronchi should then be slit open from their posterior surface and examined carefully for any evidence of erosion, ulceration, infiltration or pressure, and the sites and characters of these, as well as the positions where narrowing has taken place, should be carefully noted. For further examination of the growths, especially if they are large, I have always found it advisable to make a complete section through both lungs and the growth, in a line at right angles to the antero-posterior diameter, and extending from apex to base of each lung. In this way the general character of the growth is seen, any evidences of hæmorrhage or necroses in the central parts are noted, the relation of the vessels and bronchi is generally well made out, and the extent and general character of the invasion of the lung can be determined.

In special cases, such as hydatid cysts, aneurisms, dermoids, etc., the procedure which I have described may require to be modified, but such modifications may vary in any individual case, and the pathologist must be his own guide in the matter. He must do what he thinks best to demonstrate clearly all the leading points in the special case under consideration.

DISEASES OF THE BLOOD AND LYMPHATIC GLANDS. .

A description has already been given of the method to be employed in the systematic examination in any of these diseases, but it might aid the operator if a brief account of the essential pathological lesions in the more important of them were given.

Pernicious Anæmia.

The *skin* is often of a lemon yellow tinge, the muscles are intensely red and the fat a light yellow colour. Hæmorrhages occur in the skin and subcutaneous tissues, and also on the serous surfaces.

The *heart* is usually enlarged, pale in colour and flabby. There is extensive fatty degeneration, and this is especially seen in the muscle lying immediately under the endocardium, particularly of the left ventricle, and in the papillary muscles. The degeneration produces a mottling of the surface, and this " thrush breast " appearance should always be carefully looked for.

The *lungs* shew no special changes, though they are usually pale and may contain œdematous fluid.

The *liver* is always enlarged, of a brownish colour and very friable owing to extensive fatty changes. The cut surface should always be tested for free-iron with the hydrochloric acid and ferrocyanide of potassium test (Appendix). The distribution of the iron pigment is seen, on microscopical examination, to be confined to the outer and middle zones of the lobules, and this arrangement has been considered by some authors as specific of pernicious anæmia.

The *spleen* also shews an excess of iron which can be demonstrated by the production of the blue colour with the hydrochloric acid and ferrocyanide of potassium test.

The *lymphatic glands* shew free-iron and are usually of a deep red colour.

The *kidneys* are pale, often fatty, and also give evidence of an excess of free-iron pigment.

The *bone marrow* is increased in amount, the medullary cavity being widened. It is very red in colour, due to an erythroblastic reaction—the nucleated red cells, and particularly the large ones, being greatly increased in number.

In the *nervous system* sclerosis has been found in the posterior columns of the cord in some cases.

Chlorosis and other forms of Anæmia.

The post-mortem appearances resemble those of pernicious anæmia, but the pathological changes are usually much less marked, and some of them may be entirely absent. There is however great variation in different cases.

Leukæmia.

The *skin* is generally pale, hæmorrhages may be present, and in some cases, especially in the lymphatic type of the disease, distinct tumour-like masses may be scattered about the surface of the body.

Hæmorrhages should also be looked for in the serous and mucous membranes.

Heart. The chambers are usually filled with a clot which is of a pale or yellowish-green colour, and the muscle may be pale and fatty. Hæmorrhages into the muscles are sometimes seen.

Lungs. These shew no special changes, though large hæmorrhages may be found.

Liver. This is usually enlarged, especially in cases of lymphatic leukæmia, and frequently small whitish nodules, which must be distinguished from tubercle granulations, from areas of focal necrosis and from the nodules sometimes seen in cases of

Hodgkin's disease, are seen scattered through the substance. These are found on microscopical examination to be collections of leucocytes.

Spleen. This organ may be moderately enlarged as in the lymphatic type, or the enlargement may be very considerable as in the medullary form of the disease, weighing from five to 18 pounds. The capsule is usually thickened and large pale infarcts are frequently seen. The organ is firm, usually dark red on section, and the Malpighian bodies obscured.

Kidneys. These may shew no special changes, or they may be pale and fatty. In other cases of lymphatic leukæmia definite tumour-like masses, often with hæmorrhages into their substance, are seen projecting from the surface of the kidney.

Lymphatic tissue. The thymus usually shews no changes, but the glands in various parts of the body, the tonsils and lymphatic tissue generally may shew considerable enlargement in the lymphatic type of the disease. The tonsils should be specially examined for any evidence of ulceration or necrosis. Occasionally large tumour-like masses are found, *e.g.* in the intestine, developed apparently from the Peyer's patches or the solitary glands. It is therefore important in all cases to examine carefully the lymphatic tissue in the intestines, nasopharynx and elsewhere.

Bone marrow. In medullary or spleno-medullary leukæmia the bone marrow is pale, considerably increased in amount and semi-fluid in consistence. The medullary canal is widened owing to absorption of bone. The pallor of the marrow is due to a definite leucoblastic change, though there is also increased reaction in the red marrow. The pathologist, however, must always remember that these appearances may be obscured in old-standing cases where atrophic and degenerative changes tend to supervene. The marrow then looks translucent and gelatinous in appearance, and either pale yellow or dark red in colour. Microscopical examination should always be made.

In the lymphatic form of the disease the marrow often shews a patchy red and white appearance, due to an irregular infiltration of lymphocyte-like cells. In some cases the suggestion given is of pale, homogeneous tumours in the bone marrow.

Central nervous system. Hæmorrhages sometimes occur and may be extensive, but no other characteristic changes are described.

I have not attempted to differentiate clearly between the medullary and the lymphatic forms of leukæmia, for this must be done largely on the examination of the blood, and it is not my province in this book to deal with the purely clinical side. Every pathologist, however, must have met with types of the disease which do not in their morbid anatomy conform to one or the other of the classical forms. These intermediate cases may shew splenic enlargement and general glandular enlargement, or they may not shew general but localised glandular enlargement. These latter it is often difficult to differentiate from some of the sarcomata, and the pathologist must give his decision not from one or two apparently typical morbid changes but from the whole of the facts at his disposal.

Other Diseases of the Blood.

Purpura, hæmophilia, scurvy do not present any features which call for special examination, and though careful bacteriological examinations have been frequently made and organisms of various types isolated yet no distinct evidence of any causal relationship has been established. At the same time this should not influence the pathologist, and he should not neglect the bacteriological side of these cases.

Hodgkin's Disease (Lymphadenoma).

Lymphatic glands. Special examination should be made of the glands in the following order : the cervical, the axillary, the inguinal, and then other groups. One or more groups of these shew enlargement of the individual glands, which are usually firm and matted together by secondary inflammatory adhesions. On cutting into the glands they are seen to have a semi-translucent greyish-pink appearance and there may be areas of necrosis. Actual caseation does not occur unless there is secondary infection with *B. tuberculosis.*

The *spleen* may be considerably enlarged, but in some cases the increase in size may be very slight. The characteristic appearance is the presence of scattered, rounded or irregularly shaped whitish masses throughout the cut section of the organ. This " cold suet-pudding" appearance is very characteristic and can hardly be mistaken for any other condition by the experienced pathologist. The nodules may be very large, and in such cases there may be some difficulty in deciding whether or not the condition is one of tumour formation. Microscopical examination will usually clear up any doubt on this point

Similar nodules have been described in the lymphatic glands and in the bone marrow and should always be looked for in these situations; they are frequently present in the liver, growing in the connective tissue of the portal tract, and sometimes in the kidneys, the lungs and in the skin.

Tumours of Lymphatic Glands.

These are usually of the lymphomatous or lymphosarcomatous type, though secondary growths of sarcoma or carcinoma are common. Their examination usually presents no difficulty except in cases where the invasion is very slight and the gland, on a superficial examination, seems healthy. At a post-mortem examination on cases with malignant disease, various glands which are in the drainage area of the growth should be examined microscopically, especially if no obvious lesion presents itself on naked eye examination.

Other Lesions of Lymphatic Glands.

An examination of the lymphatic glands is very commonly neglected by the pathologist and much valuable information about the case is thus lost. Thus in chronic infective cases we frequently examine the liver and spleen for evidence of amyloid degeneration and usually neglect the lymphatic glands where the condition may alone be present, or present in a more marked degree than in the liver, spleen, etc.

Pigmentary changes are usually not of special importance, but in many cases the glands are the particular sites where pigment collects.

In all cases of tuberculosis, the glands should be specially examined, and in some cases it may thus be possible to trace the source and the method of spread of the infection. From a purely statistical point of view it is important to examine the glands in the abdomen, in the neck and in the thorax, particularly those at the root of the lung. Calcified glands are usually regarded as tuberculous, but undoubtedly in some cases tuberculosis is not the causal agent. Where possible, microscopical examination should be made of all suspicious glands and in doubtful cases an emulsion of the crushed glands inoculated into guinea pigs and rabbits.

DISEASES OF THE ABDOMINAL ORGANS.

If the systematic method of examination of the abdominal and pelvic organs and tissues, which has already been described, is followed there is little chance of any important pathological lesion being missed. At the same time it is always helpful to the pathologist in certain conditions which may be brought about by one or more various causes to have some indication of the physiological or pathological process for which he should be on the outlook. I propose, therefore, dealing with the more important of these conditions :

Hæmorrhage from the Stomach.

This very common symptom of disease may be the main factor which the clinician wishes cleared up at the post-mortem examination. The causes are various.

(*a*) *Ulceration or erosion.* The pathologist must carefully search for any evidence of *gastric ulcer* or *erosion*. The typical *peptic ulcer* can hardly be missed and all its characteristics should be carefully noted, but small *erosions* or minute superficial ulcers are very easily overlooked and especially where there has been some contraction of the musculature of the stomach after death. Only a systematic examination of the mucous membrane, with the stomach well stretched, will avoid the overlooking of some of these lesions.

My experience leads me to the view that in every case of severe hæmorrhage from the stomach a definite lesion is present in the mucous membrane of the stomach itself or of the œsophagus, and the more careful and systematic the examination is, the less will be the number of recorded cases of gastrorrhagia without a lesion of the mucous membrane.

The ulceration due to *malignant disease* of the stomach or of the œsophagus is usually very obvious, and the small erosions associated with acute gastritis and those which are present sometimes following operations in the abdomen, and particularly where the omentum or mesentery is wounded, are, in most cases, easily found. In the latter class of cases, search should be made for any evidence of thrombosis in the smaller vessels.

(b) *Passive congestion* due to obstruction in the portal system. Cirrhosis of the liver, portal thrombosis, partial obstruction of the portal vein by tumour, chronic disease of the heart and lungs, and enlargement of the spleen may lead to a distension or even to a varicose condition of the venous radicles in the mucous membrane of the stomach and particularly of those at the lower end of the œsophagus. These distended veins cause pressure and atrophy of the mucous membrane, and rupture of them gives rise to the hæmorrhage. It is often quite impossible to determine the seat of the hæmorrhage, though we know from the pathological process which has taken place that one or more definite lesion must be present.

(c) *Toxic*. Hæmorrhage from the stomach may occur in cases of septicæmia, in the specific fevers, in cases of acute yellow atrophy, in purpura, scurvy and in phosphorus and chloroform poisoning. In all these cases the hæmorrhage is due to acute degenerative changes in the smaller vessels and the lesion is not usually obvious to the naked eye. Microscopical examination, however, usually reveals the presence of marked fatty changes in the endothelium of the vessels, often over wide areas of the mucous membrane. In all such cases hæmorrhage will be found *in* the mucous membrane itself.

(d) *Constitutional or blood diseases*, such as hæmophilia and profound anæmia of any type, may have hæmatemesis as an important symptom. In such cases, microscopical examination shews the degenerative (most commonly fatty) changes in the vascular walls, though no obvious lesion may be present on naked eye examination.

(e) *Traumatic lesions* of the mucous membrane due to mechanical injuries such as external blows or wounds or internal violence by the stomach tube particularly in patients who struggle, and severe damage due to corrosive poisons are usually so obvious that they cannot be overlooked.

(f) The pathologist of course must always bear in mind that the blood found in the stomach may have come from the nose, the pharynx or the œsophagus, or from a ruptured aneurism either in the wall of the stomach or pressing on and eroding into the stomach or the œsophagus, and if he is not satisfied that the blood has come from the vessels of the stomach he must make a careful examination of any other possible site.

Dilatation of the Stomach.

The pathologist must carefully distinguish between the dilated and the displaced stomach, though in the latter there may be in addition great dilatation. According to Ewald, the maximum capacity of a normal stomach is about 1600 c.c., and measurements above this point indicate dilatation. The pathologist, however, is generally concerned with very obvious dilatation and he has to seek causes of the enlargement.

Rarely does acute paralytic dilatation come to the post-mortem table, but chronic dilatations are common and the main causes are as follows :

Narrowing of the pylorus or duodenum. The pathologist must search for any evidence of cicatrisation due to an old ulcer, of fibrous or cancerous stricture, of congenital stricture or of pressure from without by tumour or by, what is very rare, a floating or displaced kidney. Sometimes by displacement of the stomach or the liver the pylorus is dragged upon and an artificial obstruction produced. It is important, therefore, in cases of dilatation to note the position, etc. of the pylorus before the abdominal organs have been displaced.

Dilatation may be present without any obvious gross pathological cause as for example in the dilatation due to atony of the muscular coats ; to that due to repeated over-distension or to chronic catarrh of the mucous membrane, so that in many cases the pathologist may not be able to determine definitely the cause of the dilatation.

Hæmorrhage from the Intestine.

This symptom usually means that there is a very obvious lesion of the mucous membrane of the intestine, and one which can hardly be overlooked if the systematic method of examination which has been recommended is followed by the pathologist. The ulceration of dysentery, of typhoid fever and of tuberculosis of the intestine, the ulceration of colitis, duodenal ulcer and the local congestion due to strangulation or intussusception may give rise to hæmorrhage. The site of the hæmorrhage may not be very obvious in those cases which result from chronic venous congestion, profound anæmia, phosphorus poisoning and the intense congestion which sometimes follows burns of the skin, but the hæmorrhages *into* the mucous membrane are usually sufficient to determine the region from which the blood has come.

The pathologist, however, must always remember that the blood may come from the lower end of the rectum—especially from hæmorrhoids—and this area is not always carefully examined.

Diarrhœa.

The cause of this symptom may be quite evident or, on the other hand, the post-mortem examination may give little or no evidence of its cause. The pathologist expects to find intestinal catarrh but there may be no evidence of redness, swelling or increased secretion—in fact, it is rare to see the mucous membrane injected ; more commonly it is pale and covered with mucus. The pathologist, too, is sometimes led astray by changes which take place after death, such as softening and shedding of considerable areas of the mucous membrane—changes which no doubt take place more rapidly where there has been acute inflammatory changes, but which nevertheless are definitely post-mortem in most cases.

The Peyer's patches may be swollen, and very commonly the solitary lymph follicles are very prominent and frequently shew necrotic areas or follicular ulcers in the centres. Where the diarrhœa has been chronic the mucosa is usually firm and sometimes thickened and the villi and the follicles shew a slaty blue pigmentation.

The more obvious causes of diarrhœa, such as ulceration from typhoid fever, dysentery and tuberculosis and the intense enteritis of cholera, need no special reference as no careful pathologist can overlook these conditions.

Bacteriological examination of the contents of the intestine may be required and reference to the methods employed will be found in the Appendix, but for full details readers must be referred to works on Bacteriology.

Microscopical examination for fragments of mucous membrane, the ova of parasites, etc. may also be advisable, but the history and the general morbid anatomy of any given case will determine whether such an examination is necessary.

Ulceration in the Intestine.

It is sometimes important to determine from naked eye examination the nature of ulcers which are found in the intestine, and though in some cases the general morbid anatomy of the case or even the microscopical examination of the infected area may be necessary before a definite diagnosis is arrived at, yet there are some features which, if not quite characteristic, are very strong evidence in favour of one or other view. I give these briefly as a guide :

(a) *Tubercular ulcers.* These are principally found in the lower part of the ileum where the Peyer's and the solitary glands become swollen either uniformly or in scattered irregular areas, but tuberculous foci may appear in other parts of the mucous and submucous coats. The ulcers, which are at first rounded and may shew central caseation, by coalescence become very irregular. Both the floor and the edges are infiltrated and thickened—the floor appearing caseous, ragged and granular and the margin raised and irregular.

By a peripheral spread the ulcer invades the mucous membrane beyond the Peyer's follicle and may completely encircle the bowel. It also spreads deeply into the muscular and serous coats and produces in the deeper part of the serous coat numbers of tubercle granulations with often considerable thickening of that coat and adhesion to surrounding parts. With the destructive changes there are always associated proliferative ones, and the contraction of this newly formed tissue may lead to the production of strictures of the intestine. It is this proliferative change which accounts for the fact that perforation rarely occurs in tubercular ulceration.

Thus, the important points in the differential diagnosis of tubercular ulceration are the proliferative changes causing the thickened edges and floor, and particularly the presence of tubercle granulations, which can be seen in the subperitoneal tissues.

Acute tubercular ulcers which have ragged and undermined edges are rare and may simulate very closely typhoid ulceration. Perforation may occur, but usually there is evidence of well-marked tuberculosis in some other region of the intestine or in the mesenteric glands. There is usually no difficulty in diagnosis.

Tuberculous ulceration of the cæcum and large intestine is less common, tends to be more acute, and leads usually to large irregular areas of destruction of the mucous membrane. The evidence of tubercle granulations in the subserous layers of the bowels or of caseous tuberculosis in the associated glands is usually sufficient to make the diagnosis certain.

(*b*) *Typhoid ulcers.* In the early stages of the disease these are represented by irregular necrotic and ulcerated areas in the Peyer's glands and solitary follicles. The sloughs are often in position and are markedly bile-stained. At a later stage, towards the end of the third week of the disease, the sloughs separate and oval ulcers with their long axes parallel to that of the intestine are formed. The floor may be smooth or irregular and the edges are undermined. The peritoneal coat may shew very little change from the normal condition. The necrosis may have spread through the muscular coat so that the floor of the ulcer is formed by peritoneum. Perforation may have occurred, and the opening may be sealed up with a localised fibrinous exudate.

(c) *Dysenteric ulceration.* The most obvious changes are seen in the large intestine, though the lower part of the small intestine may sometimes also become involved. The ulcers at first are small, rounded and shallow, but later, by confluence, they become larger and usually oval in shape. They generally run transversely to the long axis of the bowel, have undermined edges and a floor infiltrated with inflammatory material. There is usually associated with the condition inflammatory thickening of all the coats of the intestine. The mucous membrane is often reddish or of a greenish-black colour. In some cases, large sloughs of the mucous membrane may be found. In the *diphtheritic* type the glandular tissue of the solitary glands may be almost completely destroyed, the ulcers form large, irregular sloughing areas, the submucous tissue is infiltrated with inflammatory products, and hæmorrhage is often very marked.

(d) *Ulcerative colitis.* The ulcers are usually confined to the colon though the ileum may also be involved. They vary in character, but in the most typical and advanced cases the ulceration may be very extensive so that a large proportion of the mucosa is removed.

In *Asylum dysentery* this condition is seen, but usually it extends to the large intestine and is more comparable with true dysenteric ulceration.

(e) *Follicular ulcers.* Small ulcers in the lymph follicles are common in most conditions of chronic catarrh as well as in many of the acute fevers. They have, therefore, no specific diagnostic importance.

(f) *Stercoral ulcers.* These are sometimes found especially in the large intestine above a stricture or an accumulation of solid fæces. They may be solitary, but more often they are numerous and the mucous membrane presents a " worm-eaten " appearance from the confluence of the individual ulcers. Perforation may occur. Their position behind an obstruction is usually sufficient evidence of their nature.

Abscesses in the Liver.

The pathologist will have no difficulty in recognising this condition, but he should examine carefully to determine whether the pus is in the vessels, in the bile ducts or in the liver substance itself and he should, wherever possible, trace the source of the infection.

The *solitary or tropical abscess* is usually found in the right lobe and the contents are of a brownish or reddish colour, resembling anchovy sauce, though in some cases the colour may be paler and of the consistence of cream. There may be no definite wall to the cavity or it may be surrounded by a firm, dense capsule. Microscopical examination of the contents shews that they are composed largely of broken-down liver tissue ; and the amœba of dysentery may be seen, though it can usually be better demonstrated in scrapings from the wall of the abscess cavity. Bacteriological examination should be undertaken, though in many cases the contents are found to contain no bacteria ; in others *streptococci, staphylococci* and *B. coli* may be found. Careful examination should be made of the wall to trace any evidence of perforation into the bile-ducts or into the blood vessels.

Septic and pyæmic abscesses. These are usually multiple, and in such cases the pus is very frequently found in branches of the portal vein, producing a dendritic appearance which is generally quite evident. The large portal vein and its tributaries should be carefully opened up in these cases and search made for septic thrombi, and the source of these traced to dysenteric or other ulcerative condition of the bowels, to appendicitis, to rectal affections and to abscesses in the pelvis.

Where the pus is in the bile passages search should be made for calculi, and particularly for any inflammatory or suppurative condition in the gall bladder, and for the presence of parasites.

Occasionally tuberculosis may specially affect the bile-ducts and multiple tuberculous abscesses be thus produced.

Emboli or thrombi may be found in the hepatic artery or vein or the inferior vena cava, but these conditions are extremely rare.

Echinococcus cysts may suppurate, but there is usually no difficulty is settling the diagnosis in these cases, especially if, as should always be done, a routine microscopical examination is made of the wall and contents of the abscess. The hooklets of the parasite or the laminated wall (the hydatid membrane) can generally be made out.

In all purulent conditions bacteriological examination of the pus should be made.

Acute Yellow Atrophy.

Very advanced cases of chronic venous congestion are apt to be mistaken for acute yellow atrophy, and it is therefore important to differentiate clearly between the two conditions. In both, the liver is greatly reduced in size, the capsule is wrinkled and thickened, and on section the surface is mottled— yellowish and dark-red areas being arranged irregularly. The organ may be firm in consistence, the firmness being more marked in chronic venous congestion.

Microscopical examination may be necessary before a definite diagnosis can be established between the two conditions. In acute yellow atrophy the necrosis of the liver cells is very obvious—all stages in the process can be seen ; in chronic venous congestion comparatively healthy liver cells are seen round the portal tract but the rest of the section shews dilated vessels with very thick walls and with practically no liver cells.

Suppuration in the Abdomen or Pelvis.

This may be general or local, and in either case the pathologist must search for the causal condition. The localised abscesses are most commonly subphrenic, appendicular or pelvic.

Subphrenic abscess. These most commonly arise from gastric or duodenal ulcer or from appendicitis, and these lesions are therefore first sought for. Cancer of the stomach which has destroyed the posterior gastric wall, the perforation of an hepatic or a renal abscess, an infective lesion (*e.g.* a septic infarct) in the spleen and suppuration in the pancreas or in a cyst of that organ may also be causal factors.

The pathologist must also remember that subphrenic abscesses may be secondary to infective conditions in the lungs or in the pleural cavities, and this without perforation of the diaphragm. Such a condition is sometimes found in cases of pneumonia and in pyothorax.

Appendicular abscesses. These are practically always the result of appendicitis or typhlitis and usually present no difficulty in diagnosis.

Pelvic abscesses. Not only has the pathologist to search for causal conditions as inflammation about the uterus or Fallopian tubes such as result from gonorrhœal and tubercular infections, but he has also to remember that pelvic abscesses may have their origin outside the pelvis altogether, and particularly from disease of the vertebræ and sometimes from disease in the kidney or of appendix. With ordinary care however the source of the pus is usually quite easily traced.

Addison's Disease.

Special attention in this disease is usually directed to the suprarenal glands, but in all cases the condition of the abdominal sympathetic ganglia should be investigated. In the suprarenal glands, the most usual condition is chronic tuberculosis with caseation, though fibrous atrophy of the glands may occur.

In one case which I examined the glands were represented by two blackish nodules only about the size of a split-pea, and in another case I could find no trace of suprarenal structure.

The bronzing of the skin and the other symptoms of Addison's disease may be present though the suprarenals appear healthy. In such cases it is not only important to examine the abdominal sympathetic ganglia but careful examination should be made of the tissues in the neighbourhood of the suprarenal glands, lest any condition may be present there which might interfere with the lymphatic or vascular supply of the organs.

The examination of the suprarenal glands and the neighbouring tissues should be undertaken before any of the abdominal organs have been removed.

Hæmaturia.

In cases with hæmaturia, the pathologist may have to decide whether the blood came from the kidney itself or from the urinary passages, and if the hæmaturia has been a marked symptom, it is well to remove the kidneys and urinary passages *en masse*.

In the ordinary routine examination, the kidney will be first examined and the conditions which may give rise to hæmorrhage, such as acute nephritis, renal infarction, tuberculosis of the kidney, malignant growth, the presence of calculi or of parasites, especially *Bilharzia hæmatobium*, must be carefully looked for. Under the term acute nephritis is included those congestive and degenerative changes which are associated with the acute fevers and with poisonings by turpentine, carbolic acid, cantharides, etc. The general size, consistence and colour of the kidney may indicate to the pathologist what morbid condition is present, but microscopical examination alone will enable him to give a definite diagnosis.

Aneurisms on the vessels in the kidney may rupture into the tubules. Recently I had a case of this kind, where, as a result of *polyarteritis acuta nodosa*, there were several aneurisms in the kidneys. One of these aneurisms ruptured and caused a fatal hæmorrhage.

After the kidneys have been carefully examined search is made in the ureters, in the bladder and in the urethra for the presence of calculi; for tumour, especially malignant tumour; for ulceration, especially in the bladder; for parasites; or for stricture in the urethra.

The rupture of veins in a congested mucous membrane may give rise to a considerable degree of hæmaturia, and sometimes in the early stages of enlarged prostate it may be a prominent symptom.

Again when blood is found in the urine after injuries, careful search must be made for the site from which the blood has come. Rupture of the kidney may result from a fall or a blow on the back, and the ureter, the bladder or the urethra may be lacerated in severe injuries about the pelvis. Careless catherisation, especially where a stricture is present, may cause damage and consequent hæmorrhage into the urethra.

Careful examination for the conditions mentioned above will generally reveal the cause and the site of the hæmorrhage, but a group of cases have been described particularly by Klemperer and M. L. Harris in which there was hæmorrhage and in which no causal lesion could be found.

The pathologist must carefully distinguish hæmaturia from hæmoglobinuria. Microscopical examination shews that in hæmoglobinuria the blood cells are either absent or present in insignificant numbers, and quite out of proportion to the intensity of the colour of the urine.

No special pathological lesion is usually found in the kidney, but very often the clinical history of the case makes the diagnosis quite clear.

Albuminuria.

This symptom is so generally a result of marked disease of the kidney that no difficulty, as a rule, is experienced in accounting for it. This very fact is apt to lead the pathologist into error, for it is recognised that albumen may be present in the urine without the existence of serious organic disease in the kidney.

It is not necessary to do more than mention the physiological albuminuria which may result after partaking of certain foods, the cyclic albuminuria of adolescence, and the neurotic albuminuria described by various authors. There seems little doubt that in such cases there must be some change which may be very slight and even transient, in the glomerular or tubular epithelium, but to the pathologist these changes are not sufficiently obvious to enable him to recognise them as pathological.

Febrile albuminuria. The amount of albumen which is found in the urine of patients suffering from any febrile condition is usually slight, and the pathological condition which is present during the fever, such as necrosis of the tubular cells, etc., may entirely disappear after the stage of fever has subsided. When such cases have to be examined after death the changes in the kidney may be extremely slight, or the necrosis and subsequently fatty degeneration may be pronounced.

Albuminuria associated with diseases other than renal disease.
Slight albuminuria may be associated with leukæmia, purpura,
poisoning with lead or mercury, syphilis, etc., and lesions in
the kidney may be slight or even absent. On the other hand,
in some cases of syphilis and in lead and mercury poisoning
gross changes may be found. It is important for the pathologist to remember these differences.

In epilepsy, tetanus, exophthalmic goitre, etc., albumen
may be found in the urine and the kidneys and the urinary
passages may shew no morbid changes.

*Albuminuria associated with definite lesions of the urinary
organs.* Though the lesion in the majority of cases is definite
organic disease of the kidneys—Bright's disease, amyloid
degeneration, and fatty and suppurative conditions—it must
always be borne in mind that congestion of the kidney resulting from heart disease or from pressure on the veins, and
inflammatory or suppurative affections of the pelvis, of the
kidney, of the ureters and of the bladder may be the cause
of the albuminuria.

Pyuria.

In cases in which pus is found in the urine the pathologist
must be on the outlook for the following conditions :

(1) *Pyelitis and pyelonephritis.* These conditions may be
due to the irritation of calculi, to tuberculous inflammation
or to a simple inflammatory condition, which has in many
cases spread upwards from the bladder. In all such cases
careful bacteriological examination should be made of the
purulent material, and in tuberculous cases, for a complete
diagnosis, inoculation of the pus into animals may be required.

(2) *Cystitis and urethritis.* These conditions usually cause
no trouble to the pathologist, but where they are associated
with pyelitis and pyelonephritis it may be difficult to decide
which has been the primary lesion. Where there is much
hydronephrosis, the pathologist will search for an obstruction
in the ureter or a stricture in the urethra. The former should
be searched for before the kidneys are removed, for a small
obstructing calculus may be very easily displaced or **a kink**

in the ureter straightened out during the manipulations necessary for the removal of the organs.

(3) *Rupture of an abscess into the urinary passages.*
Abscesses in the neighbourhood of the kidney may rupture
into the pelvis, the ureters or the bladder, and in examination
of these abscesses their original cause and site should be
determined.

They may be secondary to suppurative foci in the kidney
itself, in its pelvis or in the ureters, the infection spreading to
the perinephric tissues ; they may have followed suppuration
from disease of the appendix, colon or other part of the bowel ;
suppuration extending from disease, especially caries, of the
spine ; suppuration in the pleural cavity ; or they may have
been caused by damage to the intestine by blows or other
injuries.

Hydronephrosis.

Where this condition is present, the ureter and the urethra
should be carefully examined for any evidence of stricture.
In the ureter the stricture may be due to malformations, to
the presence of abnormal kinks or bends, the impaction of a
calculus, or the presence of inflammatory or tumour growth
in or around the tube. In the urethra, the most common
condition is the cicatrisation of an inflammatory mass due to
gonorrhœal infection, but a calculus may become impacted
in it. The obstruction may also be due to an enlarged prostate,
but a marked degree of hydronephrosis is not usually produced
by this pathological condition. Sections of the kidney should
be made to determine the amount of fibrous overgrowth and
the destruction of renal tissue which has taken place in these
cases.

Tuberculosis of the Kidney.

The small tuberculous granulations of an acute miliary
tuberculosis cannot be missed and need no special examination,
except that they must not be mistaken for minute abscesses.
This mistake is more liable to occur in those cases in which
the granulations have coalesced and formed wedge-shaped areas
near the surface. Microscopical examination should be made
in any doubtful case.

The more important condition for investigation is "renal phthisis" which very commonly commences in the male in the globus major of the epididymis, and spreads to involve the body of the testicle and the vas deferens. By way of the vas, the condition spreads to the urethra and bladder and up the ureters to the pelvis of the kidney. In other cases, the tuberculous process starts in the submucous coat of one of the renal pelves and spreads downward by way of the ureter to the bladder. In any given case of tuberculosis of the kidney these various sites should always be carefully examined.

Diseases of the Brain.

Cerebral Hæmorrhage.

In investigating cases of cerebral hæmorrhage it may be important to determine the exact position from which the blood has come and also the cause of the hæmorrhage. A knowledge, therefore, of the principal causes and of the positions in which the bleeding starts will be of value to the pathologist.

(1) *Extra and intradural hæmorrhages.* The majority of these result from injuries causing rupture of some of the meningeal arteries—and fractures of the skull should be carefully looked for in such cases. Minute hæmorrhages into the substance of the dura (*interstitial hæmorrhages*) may be the result of injury or may occur in cases of septic poisoning (septicæmia, scurvy, etc.) and sometimes larger ones in the membranes and intradurally are found in deaths due to infection with *B. anthracis.*

The more usual intradural or subdural hæmorrhage, "pachymeningitis hæmorrhagica," seen particularly in certain cases of insanity, epilepsy and chronic alcoholism, is characterised by a discoloration of part of the blood and especially by a delicate membranous covering which lies between the blood and the surface of the brain. The hæmorrhage in such cases comes from small degenerated vessels and is primarily a hæmorrhage into the dura ; and the membrane is a later production due to a proliferation of the epithelial lining of the dura. The clot becomes more or less organised and consequently becomes adherent to the under surface of the membrane.

Subarachnoid hæmorrhages. In these cases the blood is confined to the subarachnoid space, but may have spread very widely over the whole surface of the brain. The cause may be the rupture of a small pial vessel or an aneurism on, particularly, the vessels at the base of the brain, or it may be due to a larger hæmorrhage in the substance of the brain and which has ruptured into the lateral ventricle, passed through the foramen of Monro into the third ventricle, along the aqueduct of Sylvius into the fourth ventricle, and thence into the subarachnoid space. This blood may extend over the upper and under surfaces of the cerebellum, and to the cerebrum passing along the lines of the fissures of Sylvius or anteriorly into the longitudinal fissure over the upper surface of the corpus callosum and into the sulci on the inner surface of the hemispheres.

Sections made through the brain on the plan described on p. 118 will reveal any hæmorrhage which has communicated with the ventricles. If no internal hæmorrhage is found careful search should be made especially about the circle of Willis for any ruptured aneurism. The aneurisms are often difficult to find as the blood clot which becomes entangled round the vessels may be difficult to separate. The vessels must often be dissected from the blood clot with great care before the aneurism or the ruptured vessel is found. I have found it advantageous to strip carefully the basal vessels, separating them gently by raising the basilar artery and pulling it and its connections forward. The whole of the vessels are then floated in water and the blood gradually washed from them. In this way the aneurismal dilatation and the point of rupture may be demonstrated.

(2) *Hæmorrhage into the substance of the brain* is generally due to rupture of an atheromatous vessel or of an aneurism on such a vessel within the substance of the brain. The aneurisms vary much in size and may be microscopic. The larger ones are seen particularly on the vessels of the circle of Willis, on

the vertebral artery, on some of the internal branches of the middle cerebral, and, less commonly, on the basilar, internal carotid, posterior cerebral, anterior communicating and cerebellar. The smaller aneurisms which are specially concerned with intracerebral hæmorrhage are most common on the arterial branches which supply the basal ganglia.

More rarely, cerebral hæmorrhage is seen in acute fevers, in pernicious and other forms of anæmia, in leucocythæmia, and in phosphorus poisoning.

It is quite impossible in many cases, where the brain has been considerably torn up, to localise the vessel from which the hæmorrhage has come.

Ventricular hæmorrhage is almost invariably secondary to hæmorrhage into the substance of the brain, especially from the smaller branches of the anterior and posterior cerebral arteries—the former at the tip of the caudate nucleus, the latter at the posterior end of the optic thalamus. A rupture of an aneurism on the choroid plexus may occur. Very commonly the hæmorrhage is a large one and considerable areas of brain tissue are ploughed up, and frequently round the large hæmorrhage are seen minute punctiform hæmorrhages due no doubt to the contusion.

Hæmorrhage from the middle cerebral artery. This most commonly arises from the lenticulo-striate branch which passes to the caudate nucleus between the lenticular nucleus and the claustrum. The starting point of the hæmorrhage from this vessel is very frequently in the external capsule or the outer part of the lenticular nucleus, and the blood ploughs its way into the lenticular nucleus or even as far as the lateral ventricles.

Hæmorrhage from the anterior cerebral artery. This comes most usually from the branches which supply the anterior part of the caudate nucleus, particularly that part projecting into the lateral ventricles, and is therefore the most common source of ventricular hæmorrhage.

Hæmorrhage from the posterior cerebral artery usually comes from the branch which supplies the inner part of the optic thalamus.

Hæmorrhages in the pons and in the cerebellum. Large or small hæmorrhages may be found, those in the cerebellum being very rare.

Inflammation of the cord (Myelitis).

In the acute cases, this is generally indicated by a congestion of the vessels of the pia and a congestion and softening of the affected area which may sometimes be semi-fluid. Numerous minute hæmorrhages may be present and meningitis should always be looked for. Microscopical examination, though often yielding very little result, should always be undertaken.

In any case search should be made throughout the length of the cord for disseminated softened patches and also for sclerosed patches where there has been a proliferation of neuroglial tissue (grey softening). These areas may in many cases be found only after careful and systematic microscopical examination.

Acute anterior poliomyelitis (Infantile Paralysis).

In these cases microscopical examination alone is of value in determining the morbid anatomy of the condition. Portions of the cord, especially at the lumbar enlargement or the cervical enlargement in certain cases, should be fixed and sections made. Search of course should be made at the autopsy for any evidence of meningitis, for congestion of the pia mater, for softening, and in the later stages for any atrophy of the cord. The atrophied muscles should also be examined microscopically.

Flexner and Nogouchi have succeeded in making cultivations of small coccal-like bodies from the cord in infantile paralysis under anærobic conditions in sterile ascitic fluid containing pieces of rabbit kidney, and of reproducing the disease in animals by injections of emulsions in saline of the spinal cord. The emulsions are first filtered in vacuo under pressure. For full details reference should be made to the original papers by these authors.

Diseases of the Middle and Internal Ears.

In cases of meningitis or of cerebral or cerebellar abscess it may be advisable to open up the middle ear. In most cases it is not very important that special care should be exercised in doing this—if the chisel is placed at right angles to the petrous bone and over the roof of the middle ear and a firm blow given with the mallet, the bone will be cut sufficiently to enable the operator to remove the roof with bone forceps, and so to expose the cavity, the tympanum and the Eustachian tubes. Then with the bone forceps the mastoid antrum may be opened up by removing the bone external to the superior semicircular canal.

If a detailed examination is required of the middle and internal ears, then it is advisable to chisel carefully away the bone forming the roof of the middle ear and to open up the cavity by gradually nipping away the bone with forceps until it is well exposed. This completed, the whole temporal bone is removed and the internal ear sawn out, put into fixing and decalcifying fluids and then the semicircular canals carefully dissected out or the whole embedded in celloidin and sections made.

The skin and the superficial soft parts are reflected from the outer surface of the temporal bone, the external cartilaginous meatus being cut through close to the bone, and then with the saw a cut is made in a line joining the root of the zygoma and the apex of the anterior border of the petrous bone. A second saw cut is made posteriorly in a line joining the posterior border of the mastoid process and the foramen magnum, and the inner ends of these saw cuts joined with a chisel. With lion forceps the bone is then pulled up from its bed at its inner end and the soft parts are cut through with a knife. The squamous portion of the bone may be cut away with the saw and the remainder of the bone decalcified. For the methods used in decalcifying see Appendix, p. 222.

FOOD POISONING.

These cases may demand from the pathologist not only a post-mortem examination but in addition an examination of the infected food and a correlation of the findings in each examination.

The pathological lesions which are found at an autopsy, important as they may be from the medico-legal aspect of the case, are of very little value in determining the nature of the poison, for they are very similar whether the poisoning be caused by shell-fish, potted meat, meat pies, ice-cream, etc.

Pathological appearances. The mucous membrane of the stomach and intestine is swollen and congested, and shews minute hæmorrhagic erosions. The intensity of these reactions varies considerably, but usually they are less marked than one would expect from the severity of the gastro-intestinal symptoms. The liver, the kidneys and the spleen are usually congested, and the liver and kidneys may shew cloudy swelling or fatty degeneration.

McWeeney described in the stomach and intestine of some of his cases patches of white, prominent granules, each as large as a pin's head and containing nodules of tumid lymphoid tissue. The liver also shewed little, indistinct pale-yellowish areas or spots, which on microscopic examination were found to be due to intense fatty degeneration of the liver cells at these places.

Bacteriological examination. The contents of the stomach and intestine will probably have been submitted for examination before death; if this has not been done some of the contents are collected in sterile bottles, and careful bacteriological examination made, not only of the contents of the stomach and intestine but also of the suspected food, and similar organisms found in the various samples more closely studied.

The agglutination reactions of the various organisms isolated towards the serum of the infected individual must be tested.

It must always be remembered that bacteria may not be found in cases due purely to " ptomaine " poisoning, *i.e.* to the toxins or other products produced especially by putre-factive bacteria. With more thorough methods of examination this group of "ptomaine poisoning" is becoming considerably reduced in size.

The bacteria concerned. So many recorded cases have given " inconclusive " bacterial findings that there seems little doubt that organisms which are not at present included in the " food poisoning " group can produce gastro-intestinal irritation, but all the evidence suggests that in every case a special examination should be made in the first instance for one or more of the following organisms : *B. enteritidis, B. suipestifer, B. paratyphosus* A and B, *B. coli, B. proteus, B. botulinus.* The great majority of the epidemics which have been satisfactorily examined, both in Great Britain and on the Continent, have been shewn to be due to either *B. enteritidis* or *B. suipestifer,* therefore the first procedure will be to plate out the material to be examined on agar, on McConkey's bile salt agar, or on some other media of this class. Special colonies are picked off from these plates and examined in detail. Anærobic cultures should always be made as well as ærobic ones. Further details for the examination of these organisms will be found in text-books of bacteriology.

APPENDIX

METHODS FOR PRESERVING THE NATURAL COLOURS IN MUSEUM PREPARATIONS

In all methods it is important that the organ should be put into the preserving solution as soon as possible after removal from the body, and that washing with water before fixation should be avoided. I have found it advantageous to place the organ into the fixing fluid for a few minutes directly it is removed from the body, before its examination is undertaken, and at once to submerge any cut surface in the fluid. After this brief treatment, washing with water does not do so much harm, probably because the formalin in the solution has partially fixed the hæmoglobin in the red cells. If this method is adopted the operator may wear rubber gloves to protect his hands from the injurious effects of the formaldehyde, though personally I find that I can do this work with impunity, probably because the exposure is so short and that I immediately place my hands under running water—a procedure which I have advised in all post-mortem examinations as a means of preventing infection.

1. Kaiserling's method.

   (a) *Fixing solution :*

Formaldehyde	200 c.c.
Water	1000 ,,
Nitrate of potassium	15 grms.
Acetate of potash	30 ,,

   (b) *Developing solution :* methylated spirit.

   (c) *Preserving solution :*

Acetate of potassium	200 grms.
Glycerine	400 c.c.
Water	2000 ,,

2. Pick's method.

   (a) *Fixing Solution :*

Formaldehyde	50 c.c.
Carlsbad salt	50 grms.
Water	1000 c.c.

   (b) *Developing solution :* methylated spirit.

   (c) *Preserving solution :*

Acetate of sodium	270 grms.
Glycerine	540 c.c.
Water	900 ,,

3. Jores' solution.

   (a) *Fixing solution :*

Sodium chloride	10 grms.
Magnesium sulphate	20 ,,

Sodium sulphate   ..   20 grms.
Water   ..   ..   ..   1000 c.c.
Formaldehyde   ..   50–100 c.c.

(b) *Developing solution :* methylated spirit.

(c) *Preserving solution :*

Glycerine ⎫
Water   ⎬ equal parts.
      ⎭

4. Frost's method.

The specimens are fixed in the ordinary solutions, Kaiserling, Jores or Pick, as soon as possible after removal from the body. If much handling of the specimen is required, and especially if it has to be washed in water, it has been found advisable to place the specimen for a few seconds in the fixing solution before exposing any cut surface to the air or to water. From the fixing solution the specimens are transferred to fresh methylated spirit, in which they are kept until the natural colours have become well developed.

From the spirit the specimens are transferred directly to the following mounting fluid :

Sodium fluoride   ..   ..   80 grms.
Chloral hydrate   ..   ..   80 ,,
Potassium acetate   ..   ..   160 ,,
Cane sugar (Tate's cube)   ..   3500 ,,
Saturated thymol water   ..   8000 c.c.
Sodium chloride   ..   ..   80–100 grms.

The specimens may be put up directly in this fluid, but it is usually better to leave them in it for about a week and then transfer them to a fresh filtered solution before the final sealing up of the jars.

The colours are not only well preserved in this sugar solution, but during the first week they are rather intensified, and in many specimens where the natural colours have not been well developed in the methylated spirit, they have become much better marked in the sugar solution.

If there is much bile staining of the specimens it is well to add 10 per cent. of calcium chloride to the fixing solution

(Lorrain Smith) as the calcium salt makes an insoluble precipitate with bile pigment.

As to the advantages of the solutions, my personal experience has led me to adopt Jores' or Pick's solution in preference to Kaiserling's, and for a final mounting medium I prefer Frost's solution, though in organs which are very rich in blood it may be necessary to change the solution once or twice before the final sealing up of the jar, particularly if the specimens are large.

Among the common causes of failure to get good colour preservation are delay in putting the specimen into the fixing bath, washing with water which brings about destruction of the red cells, and imperfect fixation either by keeping the specimen in the solution for too short a period or by using the same solution for too long a period.

The period of fixation of course varies with the size and thickness of the specimen, but no harm will be done if the fixation is extended to a fortnight or with large specimens to one month. When fixation is complete the colour has been largely lost, but it is afterwards developed in methylated spirit. The development may take from half-an-hour up to six or twelve hours, but should be stopped at the point when the colour reaction is as near the normal as possible. Transference to Frost's solution at this stage usually slightly intensifies the colour.

For mounting specimens, I have found it both economical and otherwise advantageous to have special sizes of jars which take in easily half of a kidney or a slice of a given thickness of liver or other organ, of tumours, etc., so that no suspensory cords or other means of fixation are used, and that the minimum of preserving fluid is required.

Where the organ or tissue to be mounted is very small, thin or collapsible, it can be stitched on to a plate of black, white or colourless celloidin which can be purchased very cheaply, and in Frost's solution, at any rate, is quite as satisfactory as mica.

Richard Muir has recommended the embedding of the specimen in a layer of the following gelatine mixture,

and in his hands this method has proved very satisfactory :

> Thymol water (saturated in the cold)   100 c.c.
> Glycerine   ..   ..   20 ,,
> Acetate of potash   ..   ..   ..   5 grms.
> Gelatin (Coignet's gold label) ..   ..   10 ,,

Dissolve the gelatin thoroughly in the steam steriliser,
render acid to litmus with acetic acid ; clarify with white of
egg and filter.

The sealing up of Museum Jars.

(a) *With beeswax* (Frost).

(1) Thoroughly clean and dry the lid and the edges of the
jar on which the lid has to rest—these parts must be quite free
from grease ; cover these cleaned edges of the jar with melted
pure beeswax and allow this to set.

(2) Warm the lid gently and evenly in the Bunsen flame
to a temperature slightly above the melting point of the
beeswax, and place it rapidly on the ridge of wax; press
down gently, and as soon as the wax begins to set pass a hot
needle through it between the lid and the edge of the jar to
allow the heated air to escape. Allow this small aperture to
remain open until the wax has set, and then heat the air in the
upper part of the jar by gently heating the upper surface of
the lid with the Bunsen flame. Now close this small aperture
rapidly with some melted beeswax and cool down gradually
by placing a damp, cool cloth over the lid. A vacuum has
in this way been created between the under surface of the lid
and the fluid, and this aids very greatly in keeping the specimens
water-tight. When the wax has set firmly the adjacent edges
of the lid and the jar are carefully varnished with a thick *spirit*
varnish.

(b) *With elastic glue.*

For specimens mounted in sugar solution Frost recommends
that " Elastic Glue " should be substituted for beeswax—the

procedure is however the same as that used for beeswax mounting.

(This elastic glue is very cheap and is a proprietary article made by F. Collins, Little Earl Street, Soho, London, W.C.)

PREPARATIONS OF SECTIONS FOR MICROSCOPICAL EXAMINATION.

1. *Fresh material.* Small pieces of the tissue to be examined are placed in a gum-mixture for a few hours in the incubator at 37°, or preferably for 24 hours at the room temperature, and then cut on the ether or carbon dioxide freezing microtome. The sections are transferred from the razor or microtome knife to a bowl of clean water and afterwards into weak methylated spirit. From the methylated spirit they are transferred to a second bowl of water in which they straighten out, are at once floated on to slides, and pressed gently between layers of perfectly dry fine filter paper. Sections treated in this way will adhere to the slide during the subsequent manipulations for staining and mounting. Better staining results are however usually obtained by transferring the flattened out sections to a series of watch glasses containing the various staining solutions previous to fixation on the slide.

The sections are stained with any of the more suitable stains, such as hæmatein and eosin, sudan, etc. (for fat), picrocarmine, methyl-violet (for amyloid), etc.

They may be mounted in Farrant's solution or glycerine, or, in cases where the stain is not washed out by alcohol, they may be dehydrated in absolute alcohol, cleared in benzole xylol or clove oil, and mounted in balsam.

A useful gum-mixture is the following :

Gum acacia (saturated solution)	..	3 parts
Syrup (B.P.)	..	1 part
Carbolic acid	..	1 ,,

2. *Preserved tissues.* Various fixatives are used for the preservation of tissues, and the pathologist must choose the one most suitable for the work he has in hand. It is a good routine

practice to cut at least three blocks from the organ or tissue, and to fix one in Zenker's fluid, one in formaldehyde and one in methylated spirit—the Zenker's fluid is especially valuable for the preservation of nuclear figures and fibrils of all kinds; formaldehyde is valuable for the study of fat, myelin, etc.; whilst for the ordinary routine examination of tumours, and of bacteria, etc. I prefer methylated spirit.

Zenker's fluid:

Bichromate of potassium ..	..	2˙5 grms.
Corrosive sublimate ..	.. ..	5 ,,
Water	..	ad 100 c.c.
Glacial acetic acid ..	.. ..	5 ,,

The bichromate of potassium and the corrosive sublimate are dissolved in the water by the aid of heat. The proper proportion of acetic acid is added immediately before use.

The tissues, which should be cut into very small pieces, are kept in this fixative solution for from 12 to 24 hours, washed thoroughly in running water for about the same time, and then transferred to 80 % alcohol, where they may be kept until used.

Formaldehyde. The tissues are put into 5 to 10 % solution and kept in this till used.

Methylated spirit. It is generally recommended that the tissues be put into a weak solution at first, but for routine work I put them directly into the ordinary laboratory methylated spirit, in which they are kept for at least 24 hours.

Corrosive sublimate. A saturated solution of corrosive sublimate in 0˙85 salt solution is a very valuable fixing and hardening reagent. The saturation must be carried out by boiling the corrosive sublimate in the saline. On cooling, the sublimate should crystallise out. The sections are placed in this solution for 24 hours, washed over night in running water and can then be dehydrated and embedded in paraffin.

The sections before being stained should be treated with a solution of iodine in potassium iodide (iodine 1 grm., pot. iod. 2 grms., distilled water 100 c.c.) to remove any traces of the corrosive sublimate, and then washed in a very weak solution of ammonia in spirit (1 or 2 drops of liq. ammon. to 1 or 2 ounces of methylated spirit) to discharge the iodine.

Embedding in paraffin. After fixation the tissues are placed in weak alcohol, 30 % for 24 hours, and then for successive periods of 24 hours in 50, 70 and 90 % alcohol, and are then transferred to absolute alcohol for 24 hours, to equal parts of chloroform and alcohol for 24 hours, to pure chloroform for 24 hours, to equal parts of chloroform and paraffin at a temperature of about 55° for 12 hours, and then in pure paraffin for about 12 hours. The tissue is finally placed in position for cutting in a mould containing fresh melted paraffin and allowed to cool.

The process may be shortened at each stage if small blocks of tissue are used, but more satisfactory sections are obtained if the full time is given at each stage.

For rough histological diagnosis the alcohol stages can be reduced in number—the tissue is placed directly into methylated spirit and then into absolute alcohol. *Complete dehydration* is very important, and renewal of the absolute alcohol must be frequently made.

Embedding in celloidin. Where very large sections are required, or for such hard structures as skin, cartilage and decalcified bone, celloidin is to be preferred to paraffin for embedding purposes.

The tissues are completely dehydrated in alcohol, then transferred for two or three days to a solution containing equal parts of alcohol and ether. They are next placed in thin celloidin (celloidin dissolved in alcohol and ether) and afterwards in thick celloidin. In these solutions they may remain from 24 hours to three or four days, before being fixed on wooden or vulcanite blocks by the celloidin. They are allowed to dry slowly in the air and finally placed in 80 % alcohol to complete the hardening process.

Sections are cut on a sliding microtome under spirit or with the knife, which should be placed very obliquely, kept constantly wet with spirit. The sections are transferred from spirit to water and then stained by any desired method.

Rapid methods of preserving tissues. In urgent cases it may be necessary for the pathologist to give an immediate report on tissues, and rapid methods have been devised. I strongly deprecate the use of these except in very exceptional cases, for experience has proved to me how very erroneous some of these " rapid diagnoses " are.

For the application of these methods the tissues should not be more than 1 or 2 mm. thick.

1. *Rapid freezing method.* Put the tissues in 10 % formalin or in 0·85 % saline and boil for one or two minutes, place in a drop of gum or dextrin and press flat on the plate of the freezing microtome and, after freezing, cut in the ordinary way. Transfer the sections to a bowl of clean water and treat as already described on p. 210.

2. *Rapid paraffin method.* Fix a thin section of the tissue by placing in absolute alcohol for about one hour, transfer to anhydrous acetone for one hour and clear in benzol or xylol (half to one hour). Place in melted paraffin (melting point 52 to 55°) for about one hour; embed and cut in the ordinary way. If the sections are floated on to albuminised slides they may be dried rapidly and the staining process carried out in the ordinary way.

Media for the Cultivation of Bacteria.

For the routine work of the post-mortem room the following kinds of media should always be available—peptone broth, sloped agar and solidified blood serum. For the methods of preparation of such media reference should be made to text-books of bacteriology and bacteriological technique. It will be found convenient to have in addition a few tubes or plates of such special media as may be required for organisms whose immediate cultivation from the tissues is desirable and which do not grow well on the ordinary media or whose identification depends on characteristic reactions in these special media.

Gonococcus.

Serum broth or *serum agar* will be found most useful. This medium consists of ordinary peptone solution or ordinary agar, to which have been added a varying proportion of sterile serum (pleuritic fluid, hydrocœle fluid, etc.) from any of the cavities of the body.

Serum broth:

Sterile peptone broth	2 parts
Sterile serum	1 part

Tube and sterilise in the water bath at 56° C. for half-an-hour on each of five consecutive days.

Incubate tubes at 37° C. for 48 hours, and eliminate contaminated tubes.

Serum agar (Wertheimer):

Agar	2 parts
Peptone	2 ,,
Salt	0·5 part
Meat extract..	100 parts

Make reaction of media + 10. Filter, tube and sterilise as for ordinary agar. After the last sterilisation cool to 42° C. and then add to each tube an equal quantity of sterile blood serum. Slope the tubes and incubate at 37° C. for 48 hours. Eliminate any contaminated tubes.

Other methods of preparing serum agar will be found in text-books of bacteriology.

W. B. Martin recommends that for the growth of *gonococcus* that sodium phosphate should be substituted for sodium chloride in the media, and that the reaction should be 0·6 acidity to phenolphthalein.

The inoculations should be made directly from the lesion and the tubes put into the incubator at once.

Diplococcus intracellularis meningitidis. Meningococcus.

Nasgar (ascitic fluid agar) is one of the best media for the growth of this organism. The inoculation of the fluid should be made as soon as possible after withdrawal from the body, and the tubes put at once into the incubator.

Sol. 1. Nutrient agar ..   ..   ..   600 c.c.
Sol. 2. Distilled water   ..   ..   210 ,,
         Ascitic fluid ..   ..   ..   90 ,,
         Nutrose   ..   ..   ..   6 grms.
         Boil until the nutrose is dissolved.

Then add solution 2 to solution 1 which has been liquefied.
Heat in the steamer for 30 minutes, filter, tube and sterilise
as for ordinary agar (Eyre).
Boil until the nutrose is dissolved.

Diplococcus pneumoniæ and B. influenzæ.

Blood agar is the most suitable medium for these organisms—
i.e. sloped agar tubes, the surface of which has been smeared
over with fresh blood (human or rabbit), withdrawn under
strict aseptic precautions.

It is always well to incubate the tubes for 48 hours before
use, in order to eliminate any that are contaminated.

Streptococci of Rheumatic Fever.

Blood agar is a good medium for growth, but I find that
primary growths are best obtained in a fluid medium composed of equal parts of milk and nutrient broth, the mixture
being rendered slightly acid with a 10 % solution of lactic acid
as recommended by Poynton and Paine

B. diphtheriæ.

Alkaline blood serum is the most useful medium for the
primary growth of this organism from the throat, and I find
the most useful serum one to which has been added 0·7 %
of a sterile 10 % solution of caustic soda. Sheep serum is used
as it is more easily obtained than horse serum. Lorrain Smith
adds 0·15 % of sodium hydrate to fluid blood serum.

Coli-typhoid Group.

The types of media used by different workers are very
various, but for ordinary routine work I find MacConkey's
bile salt agar and Endo's medium the most useful, and I shall
give details for the preparation of these two alone.

Bile Salt Agar (MacConkey) :

1.   Emulsify 15 grms. of powdered agar in 200 c.c. of cold water.
2.   Emulsify 20 grms. of peptone in 200 c.c. of water warmed to 60° C.
3.   Mix the peptone and agar emulsions thoroughly.
4.   Dissolve 5 grms. of sodium taurocholate in 300 c.c. water, and use the solution to wash the agar-peptone emulsion into a two litre flask.
5.   Bubble live steam through the mixture for 20 minutes.
6.   Cool to 60° C. and clarify with egg.
7.   Filter, using hot-water funnel.
8.   Add 10 grms. of lactose.

It is an advantage to add 5 c.c. of a 1 % aqueous solution of neutral red.

Tube and sterilise as for ordinary agar (Eyre).

Fuchsin Sulphite Agar (Endo) :

Nutrient agar   ..   ..   ..   1000 c.c.
Lactose   ..   ..   10 grms.

Make the reaction + 3 and filter—then add

Fuchsin (alcoholic solution)   ..   5 c.c.
Sodium sulphite 10 % ; watery solution 25 c.c.

Tube and sterilise.

The Fuchsin solution is prepared as under :

Basic fuchsin ..   ..   3 grms.
Absolute alcohol   ..   ..   60 c.c.
Centrifugalise thoroughly and use the supernatant fluid.

STAINING REAGENTS.

For staining sections of tissue, in order to determine histological structure, the pathologist may use a variety of staining reagents.   I propose referring to only a few of the more usual ones which are employed in every day work.   For special stains and modifications of stains reference should be made to books of pathological and bacteriological technique, etc.

I. For *studying the histological structure of tissues* I prefer hæmatein and eosin or eosin and methylene blue.

(*a*) *Hæmatein solution*:

Hæmatein ..	.. ..	1 grm.
Absolute alcohol ..	..	50 c.c.

Allow to stand for three days until the whole of the hæmatein is dissolved, then add a watery solution of potash alum:

Potash alum	.. ..	50 grms.
Water	.. .. ..	1000 c.c.

Allow this mixture to stand for two or three weeks before use.

Eosin. A weak watery solution ($\frac{1}{8}$ to 1 %) is used, or a 10 % alcoholic solution.

The hæmatein solution is filtered on to the section and allowed to remain for five minutes or longer as it does not overstain, then it is washed off with water and the eosin filtered on and allowed to remain for one minute or longer, depending on the strength of the solution of eosin which is used. The section is now washed, dehydrated in absolute alcohol, cleared in benzole or xylol, and mounted in Canada balsam.

(*b*) *Methylene blue.* A saturated watery solution is generally employed. The section is stained first with eosin (watery or alcoholic solution) and, after washing, with the methylene blue for from one to five minutes.

A better method is that recommended by Richard Muir. The section is flooded with equal parts of a saturated alcoholic solution of eosin and distilled water, and held over the flame of a Bunsen burner; the alcohol ignites but the flame is blown out at once. This process is repeated until the whole of the alcohol has been discharged. The section is now washed and treated for five minutes with a saturated aqueous solution of potash alum, washed again and stained for one minute in a freshly prepared saturated aqueous solution of methylene blue, washed in water, differentiated and dehydrated in absolute alcohol, cleared in benzol or xylol and mounted in Canada balsam. This is a very valuable stain for demonstrating granules in the cells.

II. *For the study of bacteria in tissues or in films* the following staining solutions are most useful:

(a) *Thionin blue* in carbolic acid.

    Thionin blue ..   ..   1 grm.

    Carbolic acid (1 in 40 watery solution)   100 c.c.

(b) *Methylene blue.*

    Saturated watery solution.

(c) *Carbol-fuchsin.*

    Basic fuchsin ..   ..   1 grm.

    Absolute alcohol   ..   ..   ..   10 c.c.

    Carbolic acid (1 in 20 watery solution)   100 c.c.

This may be used either at full strength or diluted with 10 parts of distilled water.

With all these solutions the stain is applied for from half to one minute, then washed off and the film dried or the section of tissue dehydrated in absolute alcohol, cleared in benzole and mounted in Canada balsam.

(d) *Gram's stain* (modification).

The film or section is first stained with the following solution for from three to five minutes:

    Gentian violet (saturated alcoholic solution)   1 part

    Carbolic acid (1 in 20 watery solution) ..   10 parts.

This should be made up fresh at least every three days. After staining in this, the film or section is washed and then treated with a solution of iodine in potassium iodide for one minute, washed and afterwards decolourised in methylated spirit until the washings in spirit are not stained with the blue. The specimen may then be counterstained with a weak, watery solution of eosin or bismark brown, and dried or mounted in the ordinary way.

Gram's iodine solution.

    Iodine   ..   ..   ..   1 part

    Potassium iodide ..   ..   2 parts

    Water   ..   ..   ..   300 parts.

(e) *Ziehl-Neelsen's* stain for tubercle bacilli.

The section of tissue or the film is stained with carbol-fuchsin [(c) above] for one or two minutes, the slide being gently heated, washed in water, decolourised in 25 % sulphuric acid for five minutes or longer, washed thoroughly in water, treated with absolute alcohol for one minute, washed and dried if a film or dehydrated, cleared and mounted if a section of tissue.

III. *Stains for special purposes.*

(a) For *blood and bone marrow* preparations the best stains to employ are Leishman's and Jenner's. They are both eosin-methylene blue mixtures.

Leishman's method. The stain is mixed on the slide with an equal quantity of distilled water and is allowed to remain on for one or two minutes—the slide is washed with distilled water until the red corpuscles assume a salmon-pink colour, and it is then dried in the air.

Jenner's method. The slide is flooded with the stain which is allowed to remain on for a couple of minutes. It is then washed with distilled water until the salmon-pink colour of the red corpuscle is well developed, and dried slowly in the air.

These stains are also very useful for demonstrating bacteria and especially for blood-parasites such as the piroplasma, malaria, etc.

(b) For *spirochætæ*, particularly in syphilis.

(1) *Smear preparations.* The smear is to be made from the exudate of the tissue obtained by pressure and scraping. An excess of blood should be avoided.

Giemsa's method. Mallory and Wright recommend the following modification of Giemsa's method. The preparation is fixed in absolute alcohol for 15 minutes, or by heat. It is then covered with the staining solution (Giemsa staining fluid ten drops ; distilled water, to which one to ten drops of a 0·1 % solution of potassium carbonate has been added, 10 c.c.), warmed gently over the flame and allowed to cool about 15 seconds, then the diluted stain is poured off and replaced by a fresh supply which is again warmed and allowed to cool for 15 seconds. This process is repeated four or five times, after which the preparation is washed, dried and mounted in balsam. The distilled water should be added to the Giemsa staining fluid just before use.

This method may be used for staining malarial parasites, blood, etc., though when used for these purposes the potassium carbonate is not necessarily added.

Burri's Indian ink method. Equal parts of the fluid pressed from the lesion and of fluid India ink, which has been sedimented for at least a week, are mixed together on a slide, spread thinly and allowed to dry. The spirochætes remain unstained in a brown or black background.

(2) *Spirochæta in sections.*

Levaditi's method. Mallory and Wright give the following directions :

1. Pieces of tissue about 1 mm. thick are placed in 10 % formaldehyde for 24 hours.

2. Rinse in water and place in 95 % alcohol for 24 hours.

3. Place in distilled water until the tissue sinks to the bottom of the container.

4. Place in 1·5 or 3 % solutions of nitrate of silver and keep in the incubator at 38° C. for three to five days. The stronger solution of nitrate of silver is preferable for tissues removed during life.

5. Wash in distilled water and place in the following solution for 24 to 72 hours at room temperature.

Pyrogallic acid	.. ..	2–4 grms.
Formaldehyde	.. ..	5 c.c.
Distilled water	.. ..	100 c.c.

6. Wash in distilled water.

7. Dehydrate in alcohol, clear in chloroform and embed in paraffin in the usual manner.

(c) *For fat.* The sections are cut with the freezing microtome and put into 70 % alcohol. From this alcohol they are transferred to a watch glass containing a saturated solution of Sudan III or of Scharlach R. in 70 % alcohol, and are kept in this solution for about 15 minutes. They are then washed carefully in water and mounted in a watery medium, such as Farrant's solution.

Lorrain Smith recommends the use of a 2 % watery solution of Nile-blue sulphate. The sections are stained in this for five minutes, and then washed in water to which a few drops of sulphurous acid have been added.

Osmic acid may be used in 1 % solution, the sections remaining in it for two or three days and then after washing they are mounted in Farrant's solution.

Flemming's or Marchi's solutions may be used, but for details of these readers must be referred to special books on pathological technique.

(d) For *amyloid degeneration*. The sections are best cut with the freezing microtome and are stained for a few minutes, though better results are got with longer staining, in a 1 % solution of methyl-violet. The sections are then washed in water to which a few drops of acetic acid are added, and mounted in Farrant's solution or in glycerine. The amyloid is stained violet-red, the rest of the tissue blue.

(e) For *iron-containing pigment*. The sections are made in the ordinary way, either in gum or in paraffin, and are placed for from 5 to 20 minutes in a 2 % aqueous solution of ferrocyanide of potassium; and then transferred to a 1 to 5 % solution of hydrochloric acid, either in water or in methylated spirit. The sections are washed, stained, if desired, in hæmatein or saffranin, dehydrated, cleared in benzol and mounted in Canada balsam. The iron appears as bright blue granules.

Staining of Hairs for Ringworm (Frost).

1. Soak the hairs in a mixture of equal parts of absolute alcohol and ether for 15 minutes.
2. Wash in water.
3. Soak in liquor potassæ for ten minutes.
4. Wash very thoroughly.
5. Stain with Gram's anilin-gentian-violet till the whole hair appears *black*.
6. Place in Gram's iodine for five minutes.
7. Wash thoroughly.
8. Dip in methylated spirit for a second and then place on a slide in a drop of aniline oil.

9. As soon as the *hair itself* commences to decolourise transfer to the following solution for about one minute :

Aniline oil	1 part
Benzole	2 parts
Saturated solution of alcoholic eosin (filtered)	1 part

10. Wash in benzole.
11. Mount in Canada balsam.

DECALCIFYING AND FIXING SOLUTIONS FOR BONE.

The bone should, where possible, be sawn into thin slices and then thoroughly fixed in alcohol or Zenker's fluid. After Zenker's fluid the bone is washed thoroughly in water and put into alcohol for at least 24 hours.

From the alcohol the tissues are transferred to the decalcifying fluid which should be used in large amounts and frequently changed. After decalcification they are washed thoroughly in running water for 24 hours and finally hardened again in alcohol and embedded in celloidin. For decalcification nitric acid or nitric acid with phloroglucin may be used.

(1) Nitric acid—use a 5 % aqueous solution, changing the solution every day for one to four days.

(2) Nitric acid and phloroglucin :

Phloroglucin	..	..	1 part
Nitric acid	..	..	5 parts
Alcohol ..	..	..	70 ,,
Water ..	..	..	30 ,,

EXAMINATION OF FÆCES.

Microscopical examination should be undertaken for the detection of worms and their eggs—and in such cases it may be necessary to emulsify the fæces with water and to examine a series of slides of the sediment. In this way also mucus, epithelial cells, leucocytes, casts, etc. may be observed, but in some cases it may be advisable to harden the casts, etc. and make sections.

Microscopical examination too is usually sufficient for the

detection of the *entamœba histolytica* of dysentery. In such cases portions of the fæces containing mucus or blood is selected and, if the fæces are freshly passed, examination on a warm stage will be an advantage as the amœboid movements of the parasites will be detected.

For bacteriological examination an emulsion of a few loopfuls of the fæces, if they are fluid, are made in sterile bouillon, and from this plate cultures are made on suitable media. Where the fæces are solid the mass should first be emulsified in sterile water and a few loopfuls of this emulsion taken.

For special organisms suitable media must be selected—thus for *B. typhosus* the medium of Drigalski and Conradi, of Endo, or Malachite-green, for *B. coli* the medium of MacConkey, for *B. dysenteriæ* ordinary agar plates with a transference of " typhoid-like " colonies to a 1 % glucose bouillon with Durham's gas tubes, for *S. cholera* agar or a fluid media containing peptone 10 grms., sodium chloride 10 grms., potassium nitrate 0·1 grm., sodium carbonate 0·2 grm., distilled water 1000 c.c., as recommended by McLaughlin. McLaughlin also recommends that 1 gram of the fæces should be added to 100 c.c. of sterile peptone solution and incubated for six hours, before plates are made.

For further details in regard to these methods reference should be made to text-books of bacteriology.

Sterile Peptone Solution (Dunham).

Peptone	10 grms.
Sodium chloride	5 ,,
Distilled water	1000 c.c.

Heat in the steamer at 100° C. for 30 minutes.

Filter through Swedish filter paper.

Tube in quantities of 10 c.c. and sterilise at 100° C. on three successive days.

INDEX

Plague 157
rats examination of 157
Pleural cavities 31
fluid 31
Pneumococcus, cultivation of 215
Pneumonia 60, 175
interstitial 177, 178
in Sheffield grinders 179
white 60, 175
Poisoning, examination of organs 125
removal of organs 124
Poisons, acetic acid 127
alcoholism 134
alkalies 127
alkaloids 137
ammonia 127
antifebrin 136
antimony 130
antipyrin 136
arsenic 128
arseniuretted hydrogen 136
atropine 137
belladonna 137
benzene 136
bromine 134
cantharides 138
carbolic acid 137
carbon bisulphide 135
carbon compounds 136
carbon dioxide 135
carbon monoxide 135
caustic potash 128
caustic soda 128
chloral hydrate 134
chloroform 133
chloroform delayed 133
cocaine 137
copper 131
corrosive 126
creosote 137
ether 134
fungi 138
gunpowder 136
hydrochloric acid 126
hydrocyanic acid 134
illuminating gas 136
iodine 134
iodoform 134
irritant 128
lead 132
mercury 130
morphine 137
naphthaline 136
nitric acid 126
nitrobenzine 136
nitroglycerine 136
opium 137
oxalic acid 127
phenacetin 136
phosphorus 132

Poisons, potassium binoxalate 127
potassium chlorate 134
potassium nitrate 134
potassium cyanide 134
pyridine 136
resorcin 136
silver 132
strychnine 137
sulphuretted hydrogen 135
sulphuric acid 126
vegetable 137
water gas 136
zinc 131
Poliomyelitis 111, 202
Polyarteritis acuta nodosa, hæmorrhage in 195
Portal thrombosis, hæmorrhage from stomach in 186
Post-mortems, medico-legal 122
Post-mortem records 13
room, equipment of 4
Potassium binoxalate, poisoning by 127
cyanide, poisoning by 134
nitrate, poisoning by 134
Preservation of colour in specimens 205
Prostate 102
Ptomaine-poisoning 205
Puerperal fever 162
Purpura 183
Pyæmia 177
Pyelitis 197
Pyelonephrosis 197
Pylorus, stricture of 187
Pyridine, poisoning by 136
Pyuria 197

Rabies 164
Rats, special examination in plague 157
Raynaud's disease 24
Receptaculum chyli 43
Record taking 13
Rectum, examination of 97
Renal "phthisis" 199
Rheumatic fever 162
streptococci in 215
Rigidity 18
Rigor mortis 18
Ringworm, Frost's method of staining for 221
Rodent ulcer 20

Salpingitis 100
Scalp, examination of 111, 112
Scarlet fever 153
Scharlach R., for fat staining 220
Sclerosis of brain 111, 120
Scrotum, examination of 23

Printed in the United States
By Bookmasters